Substance Abuse

Editors

LESLIE H. LUNDAHL
DAVID R. ROSENBERG

PEDIATRIC CLINICS
OF NORTH AMERICA

www.pediatric.theclinics.com

Consulting Editor
BONITA F. STANTON

December 2019 • Volume 66 • Number 6

ELSEVIER

1600 John F. Kennedy Boulevard • Suite 1800 • Philadelphia, Pennsylvania, 19103-2899

http://www.theclinics.com

THE PEDIATRIC CLINICS OF NORTH AMERICA Volume 66, Number 6
December 2019 ISSN 0031-3955, ISBN-13: 978-0-323-70878-4

Editor: Kerry Holland
Developmental Editor: Casey Potter

The Pediatric Clinics of North America (ISSN 0031-3955) is published bimonthly by Elsevier Inc., 360 Park Avenue South, New York, NY 10010-1710. Months of issue are February, April, June, August, October, and December. Periodicals postage paid at New York, NY and additional mailing offices. Subscription prices are $229.00 per year (US individuals), $653.00 per year (US institutions), $315.00 per year (Canadian individuals), $868.00 per year (Canadian institutions), $345.00 per year (international individuals), $868.00 per year (international institutions), $100.00 per year (US students and residents), and $165.00 per year (international and Canadian residents and students). To receive students/resident rare, orders must be accompanied by name of affiliated institution, date of term, and the signature of program/residency coordinator on institution letterhead. Orders will be billed at individual rate until proof of status is received. Foreign air speed delivery is included in all Clinics subscription prices. All prices are subject to change without notice. **POSTMASTER:** Send address changes to The Pediatric Clinics of North America, Elsevier Health Sciences Division, Subscription Customer Service, 3251 Riverport Lane, Maryland Heights, MO 63043. **Customer Service: 1-800-654-2452 (US and Canada). From outside of the US and Canada: 1-314-447-8871. Fax: 1-314-447-8029. For print support, E-mail: JournalsCustomerService-usa@elsevier.com. For online support, E-mail: JournalsOnlineSupport-usa@elsevier.com.**

Reprints. For copies of 100 or more, of articles in this publication, please contact the Commercial Reprints Department, Elsevier Inc., 360 Park Avenue South, New York, NY 10010-1710. Tel.: 212-633-3874; Fax: 212-633-3820; E-mail: reprints@elsevier.com.

The Pediatric Clinics of North America is also published in Spanish by McGraw-Hill Inter-americana Editores S.A., Mexico City, Mexico; in Portuguese by Riechmann and Affonso Editores, Rua Comandante Coelho 1085, CEP 21250, Rio de Janeiro, Brazil; and in Greek by Althayia SA, Athens, Greece.

The Pediatric Clinics of North America is covered in MEDLINE/PubMed (Index Medicus), Excerpta Medica, Current Contents, Current Contents/Clinical Medicine, Science Citation Index, ASCA, ISI/BIOMED, and BIOSIS.

PROGRAM OBJECTIVE

The goal of the *Pediatric Clinics of North America* is to keep practicing physicians and residents up to date with current clinical practice in pediatrics by providing timely articles reviewing the state-of-the-art in patient care.

TARGET AUDIENCE

All practicing pediatricians, physicians and healthcare professionals who provide patient care to pediatric patients.

LEARNING OBJECTIVES

Upon completion of this activity, participants will be able to:

1. Review evidence for the use of contingency management in treating substance use disorders, as well as a computer-assisted delivery of substance abuse treatment.
2. Discuss the negative consequences, pharmacology, behavioral symptoms, and treatment for nicotine, alcohol, cannabis, opioid, cocaine, club, and designer drug abuse.
3. Recognize the role of prenatal alcohol and drug exposure in adolescent substance use.

ACCREDITATIONS

Physician Credit

The Elsevier Office of Continuing Medical Education (EOCME) is accredited by the Accreditation Council for Continuing Medical Education (ACCME) to provide continuing medical education for physicians.

The EOCME designates this journal-based activity for a maximum of 13 *AMA PRA Category 1 Credit*(s)™. Physicians should claim only the credit commensurate with the extent of their participation in the activity.

All other healthcare professionals requesting continuing education credit for this this journal-based activity will be issued a certificate of participation.

ABP Maintenance of Certification Credit

Successful completion of this CME activity, which includes participation in the activity and individual assessment of and feedback to the learner, enables the learner to earn up to 13 MOC points in the American Board of Pediatrics' (ABP) Maintenance of Certification (MOC) program. It is the CME activity provider's responsibility to submit learner completion information to ACCME for the purpose of granting ABP MOC credit.

DISCLOSURE OF CONFLICTS OF INTEREST

The EOCME assesses conflict of interest with its instructors, faculty, planners, and other individuals who are in a position to control the content of CME activities. All relevant conflicts of interest that are identified are thoroughly vetted by EOCME for fair balance, scientific objectivity, and patient care recommendations. EOCME is committed to providing its learners with CME activities that promote improvements or quality in healthcare and not a specific proprietary business or a commercial interest.

The planning committee, staff, authors and editors listed below have identified no financial relationships or relationships to products or devices they or their spouse/life partner have with commercial interest related to the content of this CME activity:

Sarah M. Bagley, MD, MSc; Alan J. Budney, PhD; Dana A. Cavallo, PhD; Phillippe B. Cunningham; Jeffrey L. Derevensky, PhD; Neil C. Dodge, PhD; Jennifer Ellis, MA; Jason A. Ford, PhD; Lynette Gilbeau, BEd; Emily Grekin, PhD; Staci A. Gruber, PhD; Victoria Hayman, BSc; Kerry Holland; Joseph L. Jacobson, PhD; Sandra W. Jacobson, PhD; Tamar Arit Kaminski, BS; Alison Kemp; Suchitra Krishnan-Sarin, PhD; David M. Ledgerwood, PhD; Sharon Levy, MD, MPH; Leslie H. Lundahl, PhD; Yasmin Mashhoon, PhD; Steven J. Ondersma, PhD; Rajkumar Mayakrishnan Stella M. Resko, PhD; David R. Rosenberg, MD; Sheryl A. Ryan, MD; Kelly A. Sagar, MA; Samantha F. Schoenberger; Catherine Stanger, PhD; Bonita F. Stanton, MD; Cara A. Struble, MA; Janet F. Williams, MD.

The planning committee, staff, authors and editors listed below have identified financial relationships or relationships to products or devices they or their spouse/life partner have with commercial interest related to the content of this CME activity:

Timothy E. Wilens, MD: consultant/advisor for Alcobra Ltd, Kempharm, Inc., Otsuka America Pharmaceutical, Inc., and Ironshore, Inc.; receives royalties from Guilford Press, Cambridge University Press, and Elsevier.

UNAPPROVED/OFF-LABEL USE DISCLOSURE

The EOCME requires CME faculty to disclose to the participants:

1. When products or procedures being discussed are off-label, unlabelled, experimental, and/or investigational (not US Food and Drug Administration [FDA] approved); and
2. Any limitations on the information presented, such as data that are preliminary or that represent ongoing research, interim analyses, and/or unsupported opinions. Faculty may discuss information about pharmaceutical agents that is outside of FDA-approved labelling. This information is intended solely for CME and is not intended to promote off-label use of these medications. If you have any questions, contact the medical affairs department of the manufacturer for the most recent prescribing information.

TO ENROLL

To enroll in the *Pediatric Clinics of North America* Continuing Medical Education program, call customer service at 1-800-654-2452 or sign up online at http://www.theclinics.com/home/cme. The CME program is available to subscribers for an additional annual fee of USD 301.60.

METHOD OF PARTICIPATION

In order to claim credit, participants must complete the following:

1. Complete enrolment as indicated above.
2. Read the activity.
3. Complete the CME Test and Evaluation. Participants must achieve a score of 70% on the test. All CME Tests and Evaluations must be completed online.

In order to claim MOC points, participants must complete the following:

1. Complete steps listed above for claiming CME credit
2. Provide your specialty board ID#, birth date (MM/DD), and attestation.
3. Online MOC submission is only available for the American Board of pediatrics' (ABP) Maintenance of Certification (MOC) program

CME INQUIRIES/SPECIAL NEEDS

For all CME inquiries or special needs, please contact elsevierCME@elsevier.com

Contributors

CONSULTING EDITOR

BONITA F. STANTON, MD
Founding Dean, Hackensack Meridian School of Medicine at Seton Hall University, President, Academic Enterprise, Hackensack Meridian Health Robert C. and Laura C. Garrett Endowed Chair for the School of Medicine, Professor of Pediatrics, Nutley, New Jersey, USA

EDITORS

LESLIE H. LUNDAHL, PhD
Associate Professor, Substance Abuse Research Division, Department of Psychiatry and Behavioral Neurosciences, Wayne State University School of Medicine, Detroit, Michigan, USA

DAVID R. ROSENBERG, MD
Professor and Chair, Department of Psychiatry and Behavioral Neurosciences, Wayne State University School of Medicine, Detroit, Michigan, USA

AUTHORS

SARAH M. BAGLEY, MD, MSc
Clinical Addiction Research and Education Unit, Section of General Internal Medicine, Department of Medicine, Division of General Pediatrics, Department of Pediatrics, Boston University School of Medicine, Boston Medical Center, Grayken Center for Addiction, Boston, Massachusetts, USA

ALAN J. BUDNEY, PhD
Professor, Department of Psychiatry, Center for Technology and Behavioral Health, Geisel School of Medicine at Dartmouth, Lebanon, New Hampshire, USA

DANA A. CAVALLO, PhD
Assistant Professor, Department of Psychiatry, Yale School of Medicine, New Haven, Connecticut, USA

PHILLIPPE B. CUNNINGHAM, PhD
Department of Psychiatry and Behavioral Sciences, Division of Global and Community Health, Family Services Research Center, Medical University of South Carolina, Charleston, South Carolina, USA

JEFFREY L. DEREVENSKY, PhD
James McGill Professor, Director, International Centre for Youth Gambling Problems and High-Risk Behaviors, McGill University, Montreal, Quebec, Canada

NEIL C. DODGE, PhD
Research Associate, Department of Psychiatry and Behavioral Neurosciences, Wayne State University School of Medicine, Detroit, Michigan, USA

JENNIFER D. ELLIS, MA
Doctoral Student, Departments of Psychiatry and Behavioral Neurosciences, and Psychology, Wayne State University, Detroit, Michigan, USA

JASON A. FORD, PhD
Associate Professor of Sociology, University of Central Florida, Orlando, Florida, USA

LYNETTE GILBEAU, BEd
International Centre for Youth Gambling Problems and High-Risk Behaviors, McGill University, Montreal, Quebec, Canada

EMILY GREKIN, PhD
Associate Professor and Associate Chair, Department of Psychology, Wayne State University, Detroit, Michigan, USA

STACI A. GRUBER, PhD
Associate Professor, Department of Psychiatry, Harvard Medical School, Boston, Massachusetts, USA; Director, Cognitive and Clinical Neuroimaging Core, Director, Marijuana Investigations for Neuroscientific Discovery, McLean Hospital, McLean Imaging Center, Belmont, Massachusetts, USA

VICTORIA HAYMAN, BSc
International Centre for Youth Gambling Problems and High-Risk Behaviors, McGill University, Montreal, Quebec, Canada

JOSEPH L. JACOBSON, PhD
Distinguished Professor, Department of Psychiatry and Behavioral Neurosciences, Wayne State University School of Medicine, Detroit, Michigan, USA

SANDRA W. JACOBSON, PhD
Distinguished Professor, Department of Psychiatry and Behavioral Neurosciences, Wayne State University School of Medicine, Detroit, Michigan, USA

TAMAR ARIT KAMINSKI, BS
Clinical Research Coordinator, Pediatric Psychopharmacology Program, Division of Child Psychiatry, Massachusetts General Hospital, Boston, Massachusetts, USA

SUCHITRA KRISHNAN-SARIN, PhD
Professor, Department of Psychiatry, Yale School of Medicine, New Haven, Connecticut, USA

DAVID M. LEDGERWOOD, PhD
Department of Psychiatry and Behavioral Neurosciences, Wayne State University, Detroit, Michigan, USA

SHARON LEVY, MD, MPH
Adolescent Substance Use and Addiction Program, Division of Developmental Medicine, Department of Pediatrics, Boston Children's Hospital, Center for Adolescent Substance Abuse Research, Division of Adolescent and Young Adult Medicine, Boston Children's Hospital, Boston, Massachusetts, USA

LESLIE H. LUNDAHL, PhD
Associate Professor, Substance Abuse Research Division, Department of Psychiatry and Behavioral Neurosciences, Wayne State University School of Medicine, Detroit, Michigan, USA

YASMIN MASHHOON, PhD
Assistant Professor, Department of Psychiatry, Harvard Medical School, Boston, Massachusetts, USA; Neuroscientist, Behavioral Psychopharmacology Research Laboratory, McLean Imaging Center, Mclean Hospital, Belmont, Massachusetts, USA

STEVEN J. ONDERSMA, PhD
Professor, Department of Psychiatry and Behavioral Neurosciences, Deputy Director, Merrill Palmer Skillman Institute, Wayne State University, Detroit, Michigan, USA

STELLA M. RESKO, PhD
Associate Professor, School of Social Work and Merrill Palmer Skillman Institute, Wayne State University, Detroit, Michigan, USA

SHERYL A. RYAN, MD
Professor of Pediatrics, Chief, Division of Adolescent Medicine, Department of Pediatrics, Milton S. Hershey Medical Center, Penn State Hershey Children's Hospital, Hershey, Pennsylvania, USA

KELLY A. SAGAR, MA
Research Associate, Department of Psychiatry, Harvard Medical School, Boston, Massachusetts, USA; Cognitive and Clinical Neuroimaging Core, Marijuana Investigations for Neuroscientific Discovery, McLean Hospital, McLean Imaging Center, Belmont, Massachusetts, USA

SAMANTHA F. SCHOENBERGER, BA
Clinical Addiction Research and Education Unit, Section of General Internal Medicine, Department of Medicine, Boston University School of Medicine, Boston Medical Center, Boston, Massachusetts, USA

CATHERINE STANGER, PhD
Associate Professor, Department of Psychiatry, Center for Technology and Behavioral Health, Geisel School of Medicine at Dartmouth, Lebanon, New Hampshire, USA

CARA A. STRUBLE, MA
Departments of Psychiatry and Behavioral Neurosciences, and Psychology, Wayne State University, Detroit, Michigan, USA

TIMOTHY E. WILENS, MD
Chief, Child & Adolescent Psychiatry, Massachusetts General Hospital, Professor of Psychiatry, Harvard Medical School, Boston, Massachusetts, USA

JANET F. WILLIAMS, MD
Vice Dean for Faculty, Department of Pediatrics, Long School of Medicine, Professor of Pediatrics, Distinguished Teaching Professor, University of Texas Health San Antonio, San Antonio, Texas, USA

Contents

Section 1: Drug Abuse

> Rates of certain tobacco products have decreased over the past decade, but nicotine use disorder is still prevalent among adolescents. New trends in tobacco use, such as in the use of electronic cigarettes, are creating alarm. This article reviews nicotine addiction and measurement in adolescents, along with potential health risks and comorbidities. Various psychosocial and pharmacologic interventions are reviewed along with novel interventions that show promise for reducing tobacco use in this vulnerable population.

> Alcohol use during adolescence is an important and modifiable health risk behavior given the significant acute consequences and long-term impacts on the developing brain. Alcohol is the most common substance used by young adults 12 to 17 years old, with binge drinking, polysubstance use, and co-occurring mental health disorders posing particular concerns in this age group. Physicians can play a crucial role in screening and responding to alcohol use, with targeted brief interventions designed to delay or decrease use.

> As an increasing number of states legalize cannabis use for recreational and/or medical purposes, it is increasingly important to understand the neural and cognitive consequences of recreational cannabis use in adolescent consumers. Adolescence is marked by ongoing neuromaturational processes, making this a particularly vulnerable period, particularly regarding exposure to drugs, including cannabis. This review highlights evidence from studies documenting the neural impact of cannabis use in adolescence and explores mediating factors related to cannabis use.

Cannabis continues to be the most widely used illicit substance among youth, as many teens view the risks of cannabis consumption to be low. With cannabis laws becoming lax and dispensaries more prevalent throughout the United States, highly concentrated Δ-9-tetrahydrocannibinol (THC) is widely available. This article examines the available literature on consumption of concentrated THC, focusing on potential consequences of concentrate use among youth. Various methods for consuming concentrated THC, including ingestion of edibles, vaping, and dabbing are discussed, along with associated risks of each consumption method. Recommendations for health professionals are provided.

Although recent spikes in overdose deaths are largely attributable to heroin and fentanyl, prescription opioids still account for a significant percentage of overdose deaths. Additionally, overdose deaths are not a problem solely for adults; roughly 8% of all overdose deaths occur in persons aged 15 to 24. In addition to identifying factors that increase risk for misuse and negative outcomes among adolescents, research must examine the causal mechanisms that link these factors to increased risk. Finally, the extant research must serve as the foundation for prevention/intervention strategies and identify treatments that are effective among adolescents with opioid use disorders.

The nonmedical use of prescription stimulants has become increasingly pervasive among transitional age youth (TAY), aged 16 years to 26 years. Although therapeutically administered stimulants are regarded as safe and effective in TAY with attention-deficit/hyperactivity syndrome (ADHD), stimulant misuse is of concern due to prevalence, behavioral health and substance use correlates, and negative short-term and long-term outcomes. Although academic motivations primarily drive misuse, it is unclear whether prescription ADHD stimulants enhance cognition. Providers are advised to exercise precautions when prescribing ADHD medications, enhance surveillance for misuse, and screen those with misuse for ADHD and other psychopathology, executive dysfunction, and substance use disorders.

Club drugs and "other" abusable substances are briefly overviewed as a reminder about the wide variety of known and unknown substances used by adolescents, the high potential for direct and interactive substance use effects to manifest acutely and chronically, and the vigilance needed to anticipate and recognize the new effects and drug-drug interactions arising as novel substances continue to be custom "designed," manufactured, and marketed to meet substance use trends. This article discusses dextromethorphan, flunitrazepam (Rohypnol), gamma-hydroxybutyrate, inhalants, ketamine, lysergic acid diethylamide, methylenedioxymethamphetamine, phencyclidine, Salvia divinorum (salvia), synthetic cannabinoids, and synthetic cathinones (bath salts).

Sheryl A. Ryan

Cocaine use by adolescents and young adults continues to be a significant public health issue and the cause of medical and psychological morbidity and mortality. Although use rates are lower than those seen with alcohol, tobacco, and other illicit substances such as marijuana, cocaine is highly addictive and presents significant acute and long-term medical and psychological effects. This article reviews the epidemiology of cocaine use among adolescents and young adults, discusses the pharmacology and neurobiology of cocaine use and dependence, provides information regarding acute intoxication and systemic effects seen with more chronic use, and describes current assessment and treatment approaches.

Section 2: Special Topics

Neil C. Dodge, Joseph L. Jacobson, and Sandra W. Jacobson

Prenatal exposure to alcohol and drugs is associated with physical, cognitive, and behavioral problems across the offspring's lifespan and an increased risk of alcohol and drug use in adolescent and young adult offspring. These prenatal effects continue to be evident after control for demographic background and parental alcohol and drug use. Behavior problems in childhood and adolescence associated with prenatal exposures may serve as a mediator of the prenatal exposure effects on offspring substance use.

Jeffrey L. Derevensky, Victoria Hayman, and Lynette Gilbeau

The introduction of behavioral addictions is a relatively new concept in psychiatry. It was not until 2010 that the term behavioral addictions was added to the official classification of psychiatric diagnoses in the Diagnostic and Statistical Manual of Mental Disorders, Fifth Edition. Gambling, typically thought to be an adult behavior, has become commonplace among adolescents. Although technological advances have made accessing information and communication easier, excessive use of the Internet and smartphones can result in multiple mental and physical health issues. Gambling disorders, gaming disorders, Internet use disorder, and excessive smartphone use often begin during childhood and adolescence.

PEDIATRIC CLINICS OF NORTH AMERICA

SERIES OF RELATED INTEREST

Clinics in Perinatology
https://www.perinatology.theclinics.com/
Advances in Pediatrics
https://www.advancesinpediatrics.com/

Foreword

Substance Abuse in the United States: It's Not New News

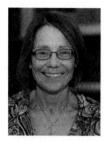

Bonita F. Stanton, MD
Consulting Editor

This issue of *Pediatric Clinics of North America* is devoted to adolescent substance abuse. Adolescence has long been recognized as the developmental period associated with experimentation across a vast array of behaviors, including substance use. Accordingly, substantial literature has been (and remains) committed to adolescent substance abuse; a PubMed search of the published literature reveals that, over the last 10 years, 7841 publications, and over the last 5 years, 3146 publications, have addressed adolescent drug use.

Substance use among the general population, including adolescents, is not a new phenomenon in the United States. Rather, it appears to have been part of our history since the colonial days. Throughout the 1800s, the medical profession was unwittingly involved in developing opioid and alcohol dependence by using these substances to reduce pain during surgical procedures and to treat injuries due to war, work, and accidents. At that time, the addictive qualities of opium were not fully understood. During the 1800s, cocaine, morphine, and codeine were introduced, again with little appreciation of the consequences of their use. It was during the Civil War that the addictive nature of these drugs began to be appreciated, although throughout the rest of the century, these drugs remained largely unregulated.[1]

As it became clearer that the drugs were a serious problem, regulations were developed, and legislation was approved to help contain the problem. In 1906, 1914, and 1918, a series of legislative initiatives were passed establishing regulations for the use of these drugs and treatment options for those addicted.

Despite this long experience with drugs, it was not until the 1960s that "recreational drug use" emerged, and has remained a major problem among teens since then. The popularity of specific drugs has varied considerably throughout the last 50 years. Beginning in the 1960s and 1970s, substantially more funding has been directed toward rehabilitation and prevention.[1,2] There remains considerable variation in the

https://doi.org/10.1016/j.pcl.2019.08.016
0031-3955/19/© 2019 Published by Elsevier Inc.
pediatric.theclinics.com

use of specific drugs; for example, rates of marijuana use have varied greatly.[2,3] A recent phenomenon has been the use of "vaping devices" with the possibility that there is concern not only about the drugs being vaped but also about the "vaping" process itself. Drug use is highest among persons in their late teens and early twenties.[3]

This issue represents a thoughtful and thorough state-of-the-art update on a range of currently abused drugs, the epidemiology of substance use, and promising new treatment approaches. I believe that all health care providers responsible for adolescents will find the articles in this issue of *Pediatric Clinics of North America* to be relevant and interesting.

Bonita F. Stanton, MD
Hackensack Meridian School of Medicine
at Seton Hall University
340 Kingsland Street, Building 123
Nutley, NJ 07110, USA

E-mail address:
bonita.stanton@shu.edu

REFERENCES

1. A forever recovery. The history of drug abuse in the United States. Available at: https://aforeverrecovery.com/blog/drug-abuse/the-history-of-drug-abuse-in-the-united-states/. Accessed September 4, 2019.
2. National Institutes of Health: National Institute on Drug Abuse. Teens using vaping devises in record numbers. Available at: https://www.drugabuse.gov/news-events/news-releases/2018/12/teens-using-vaping-devices-in-record-numbers. Accessed September 4, 2019.
3. National Institutes of Health: National Institute on Drug Abuse. Advancing addiction science: nationwide trends. Available at: https://www.drugabuse.gov/publications/drugfacts/nationwide-trends. Accessed September 4, 2019.

Preface

Adolescent Substance Abuse and Treatment: A Primer for Clinicians

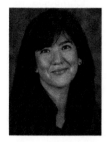 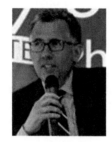

Leslie H. Lundahl, PhD   David R. Rosenberg, MD
Editors

Substance use and abuse by adolescents continue to be a major public health concern. According to the most recent Monitoring the Future survey, by senior year in high school, about 60% of teens will have tried alcohol; almost 50% will have smoked marijuana; and about 16% will have used a prescription medication for a nonmedical reason.

The teenage years are a critical period during which the developing brain is highly vulnerable to exposure to drugs of abuse, which can interfere with normal brain maturation and lead to potentially lifelong cognitive and socioemotional consequences. Most substance use initiation occurs during adolescence and young adulthood, and earlier initiation of substance use is an important predictor of developing a substance use disorder later in life. Thus, early identification of and intervention for problematic substance use are of paramount importance.

Clinicians who care for adolescents and young adults who use and/or misuse psychoactive substances need to stay abreast of shifting attitudes toward and patterns of drug use, so they can recognize problems as they occur and offer appropriate intervention. However, clinicians often report they do not feel comfortable asking about drug and alcohol use, generally because they lack familiarity with drugs, their street names, and their effects. Drug formulations and methods of use can change rapidly, and youth are often at the vanguard of these shifts. This issue was designed to assist clinicians who work with adolescents to feel more confident having conversations about drugs with their patients, and to provide a broader understanding of factors involved in substance use and intervention.

The first article addresses nicotine use disorders in adolescents and includes important information about the potential dangers of vaping and the use of e-cigarettes, which have become extremely common in youth. Alcohol remains the most widely used psychoactive substance among adolescents, and the second article surveys

Pediatr Clin N Am 66 (2019) xvii–xix
https://doi.org/10.1016/j.pcl.2019.08.015
0031-3955/19/© 2019 Published by Elsevier Inc.

alcohol use disorders in addition to binge drinking and polysubstance use. The issue's third article presents data on cognitive consequences of cannabis use, a particularly timely discussion given the changing legal landscape around marijuana use, as well as the increasing perception among adolescents that marijuana is harmless. We then learn about highly potent THC (tetrahydrocannabinol) "concentrates," which are often consumed (edibles) or inhaled through a process of vaping or "dabbing." Unfortunately, adolescents and young adults have not escaped the current opioid epidemic, and the article that follows describes both medical and nonmedical use of opioids in this vulnerable population. Clinicians who work with high school and college students are familiar with the use of psychostimulants as study aids, or cognitive enhancers. This topic is discussed, and recent studies examining whether these medications improve cognitive functioning in youth without attention-deficit/hyperactivity disorder are presented in the issue's next article. The issue then provides an update on club, designer, and "other" drugs, including MDMA/molly, ketamine, inhalants, and LSD, which continue to be popular among adolescents and young adults who frequent clubs and music festivals. Finally, use and consequences of cocaine and crack cocaine are presented in the last article of this section of the issue.

The issue then shifts from specific drugs of abuse to special current topics in the adolescent substance abuse literature. The first article in the section, Effects of Fetal Substance Exposure on Offspring Substance Use, examines the role of prenatal alcohol and drug exposure in adolescent substance use. This is followed by a discussion of behavioral addictions, including problematic gambling, gaming, Internet, and smartphone use. The article that follows is a review of evidence for the use of contingency management, which has shown promise in treating substance use disorders. The theory behind and evidence for the efficacy of juvenile drug courts to address substance use and conduct disorders are examined in the second to last article before the issue concludes with a discussion about a highly relevant mode of treatment for a tech-savvy population: computer-assisted delivery of substance abuse treatment.

This issue brings together diverse perspectives on a broad range of topics that are important in the area of adolescent and young adult substance use. Each article introducing specific drugs of abuse focuses on the negative consequences of addiction and presents information on pharmacology, behavioral symptoms, and treatment for each substance. Novel approaches to intervention, behavioral addictions, and substance use associated with prenatal alcohol and drug exposure also are discussed.

We are indebted to the authors, who generously submitted their work for this special issue. Everyone who was asked to contribute did so with enthusiasm and great attention to detail, and we thank them for their diligence and insights. Working with adolescents is challenging, often frustrating, but always important and fascinating. We hope that all clinicians who encounter and address psychoactive substance use/abuse among adolescents are informed and motivated by these excellent contributions.

ACKNOWLEDGMENTS

The editors gratefully acknowledge support from the Helene Lycaki/Joe Young, Sr. funds from the State of Michigan.

Leslie H. Lundahl, PhD
Substance Abuse Research Division
Department of Psychiatry and
Behavioral Neurosciences
Wayne State University School of Medicine
3901 Chrysler Service Drive, Suite 2A
Detroit, MI 48201, USA

David R. Rosenberg, MD
Department of Psychiatry and
Behavioral Neurosciences
Wayne State University School of Medicine
3901 Chrysler Service Drive, Suite 2A
Detroit, MI 48201, USA

E-mail addresses:
llundahl@med.wayne.edu (L.H. Lundahl)
drosen@med.wayne.edu (D.R. Rosenberg)

Section 1: Drug Abuse

Nicotine Use Disorders in Adolescents

Dana A. Cavallo, PhD*, Suchitra Krishnan-Sarin, PhD

KEYWORDS

• Adolescent • Nicotine • Tobacco • Tobacco treatment

KEY POINTS

- Novel tobacco products, such as e-cigarettes, have produced increased rates of nicotine use among youth.
- Several empirically supported psychosocial, pharmacologic, and innovative interventions exist.
- Despite advances in the treatment of nicotine use disorders in adolescents, many challenges persist.

INTRODUCTION

Tobacco use, which is initiated and established primarily during adolescence, remains a significant public health concern. Recent evidence from the Centers for Disease Control and Prevention's National Youth Tobacco Survey indicated that about 27% of high schoolers and 7% of middle schoolers report current use of tobacco, with many youth using 2 or more types of tobacco products.[1] Cigarette smoking rates have declined over the past decade, with past 30-day smoking at about 8% for high schoolers and 2% for middle schoolers, and rates of cigar/cigarillo, hookah, and smokeless tobacco use have also decreased or remained steady.[2]

Although use rates of certain tobacco products have decreased over the past decade, new trends, such as the use of electronic cigarettes, are creating alarm. E-cigarettes are battery-operated devices that contain nicotine, flavorings, and other chemicals.[3] E-cigarettes and vaping have gained popularity with adolescents over the past decade, especially with the introduction of podlike devices. In 2019, past 30-day vaping was reported by 21% of high schoolers and 5% of middle schoolers, an increase of about 1.5 million youth in 1 year.[1]

Today's popular tobacco products are more enticing than ever before, with design and innovation,[4] as well as flavorings,[5] making these products very appealing to

No financial conflicts of interest.
Yale School of Medicine, SAC, 34 Park Street, New Haven, CT 06519, USA
* Corresponding author.
E-mail address: Dana.Cavallo@yale.edu

youth. E-liquids contain more than 15,000 flavors,[6] and flavored cigars/cigarillos and hookah are also very popular, with 73% of high school students and 56% of middle school students reported using a flavored tobacco product in the past 30 days.[7] Although e-cigarettes are being proposed as a harm-reduction strategy for combustible tobacco users seeking to quit, regulatory efforts on e-cigarettes need to find a way to reduce their appeal to youth to reduce nicotine addiction and the risk of progressing to combustible tobacco use.

NICOTINE AND ADDICTION

Although the landscape of tobacco use has changed in adolescents, nicotine remains the common addictive ingredient in these products. Nicotine is a central nervous stimulant that binds to the nicotinic acetylcholine receptors in the brain,[8] which is followed by the subsequent release of dopamine, signaling a pleasurable experience.[9] Nicotine is highly addictive and leads to withdrawal symptoms upon cessation of use, which may include irritability, anxiety, and craving for nicotine.

Nicotine's effects are related to the dose of nicotine as well as to its rate of delivery. For example, nicotine delivery from combustible products that are inhaled and rapidly achieve high blood nicotine levels is much more reinforcing than slower delivery from products like the transdermal nicotine patch and nicotine gum. The issue of nicotine delivery has become more complicated by the recent availability of e-cigarette systems with nicotine salts (like the JUUL). Although much more needs to be learned about these products, it has been suggested that nicotine salts have a smoother throat hit than freebase nicotine (which is used in most combustible tobacco products), and that this smoother taste allows users to vape higher levels of nicotine comfortably, which could lead to greater nicotine addiction.

Some other features of tobacco products that enhance their addictive potential among youth include the ease of access and cultural acceptance of these products, the social and behavioral rewards, and the cues associated with tobacco use. Youth are conditioned to use tobacco products in specific situations, such as after a meal, with an alcoholic drink, or with friends who smoke, and these associations repeated many times cause the environmental situations to become powerful cues. Similarly, aspects of the drug-taking process, such as the taste or feeling, become connected with the pleasurable effects of smoking.

Nicotine dependence is common in adults, but it is also a reality for adolescents, with the onset of dependence on combustible products occurring very soon after initiation of smoking.[10] Existing evidence suggests that youth are sensitive to nicotine and experience nicotine dependence sooner than adults.[11] The *Diagnostic and Statistical Manual of Mental Disorders* (Fifth Edition) identifies a diagnosis of Tobacco Use Disorder in those who are dependent on nicotine owing to the use of tobacco products. Youth who use multiple tobacco products are at higher risk for developing nicotine dependence and may be more likely to continue tobacco use as adults.

MEASUREMENT

Various objective measures exist to biochemically verify tobacco use.[12] Breath carbon monoxide (CO) is useful for determining smoking status, but its short half-life limits its sensitivity and specificity. Given the short half-life of nicotine (approximately 2 hours), a metabolite of nicotine, cotinine, is often measured in blood, saliva, or urine and is highly specific and sensitive for measuring tobacco use behaviors, when nicotine replacement therapy (NRT) is not used. Finally, anabasine and anatabine are 2 nicotine-related alkaloids present in tobacco that can be measured if NRTs are used.[13]

Some popular self-report measures of nicotine dependence in adolescents include the modified Fagerstrom Tolerance Questionnaire[14] (mFTQ), the Hooked on Nicotine Checklist,[15] and the Autonomy Over Tobacco Scale.[16] The self-report mFTQ is an appealing measure because of its widespread use, quantitative determination of nicotine dependence, and validation with objective biochemical data (ie, salivary cotinine levels).[17] Although most of these measures have been revised to assess e-cigarette dependence,[18] new measures specific to electronic cigarette use and dependence are being modified and developed.[19]

Discrepancies between biological indicators and self-report exist and may be higher among adolescents than adults, with studies suggesting that adolescents may underreport or overreport their tobacco use,[20] although 1 study of self-report verified biochemically suggested reliability.[21] Some suggested correlates of inconsistency include self-reported parental smoking, perceived smoking by peers, exposure to passive smoke, and psychosocial variables, as well as the conditions of the interview setting.[20]

HEALTH RISKS OF TOBACCO PRODUCTS

Early onset of tobacco use is associated with increased incidence of health problems during adulthood, such as heart disease, lung disease, and cancer, as well as an increased susceptibility to a variety of infections, a reduced sensitivity to insulin, and an increased onset of diabetes.[8] Furthermore, exposure to nicotine may induce critical changes in brain circuitry related to learning, memory, and mood.[22] Because adolescence is known to be a "critical period" of brain development, genetic changes induced by tobacco carcinogens may increase susceptibility to the harmful impact of continued tobacco use.[23]

Although much is known about the short-term and long-term effects of combustible and oral tobacco products, little is known about the health risks of e-cigarettes. E-juice contains propylene glycol and vegetable glycerin, which are known to be respiratory irritants.[24] E-cigarettes may contain metallic particles, such as chromium, cadmium, or lead, that are discharged from heating coils and may create toxic effects on vital organs.[25] Furthermore, the flavors in e-liquids are created using chemicals, which are also present in cigarettes and are known to cause inflammation.[26]

COMORBIDITIES

Tobacco addiction is much more prevalent in people with mental illness and substance use disorders[27] and, among youth, there is a strong relationship between smoking and depression, anxiety, and stress.[28] One mechanism thought to underlie comorbid nicotine addiction with mental health disorders is a shared genetic susceptibility.[29] Also, nicotine may serve to medicate some psychiatric symptoms, enhance cognitive deficits in youth with attention-deficit/hyperactivity disorder[30] as well as reduce unpleasant sedating side effects of psychiatric medications, providing additional motivations for tobacco use. The adverse health consequences of tobacco use in those with comorbid mental illness and substance use disorders are considerable, often leading to premature death from cardiovascular disorders and diabetes.[31]

Another concern about tobacco use disorders is the gateway effect. An association between cigarette smoking and future substance use has been shown,[32] suggesting that adolescents who are exposed to nicotine are more likely to go on to use marijuana and alcohol. Similar relationships are also emerging with the use of e-cigarettes. For example, adolescents who use e-cigarettes are more likely to try other types of tobacco, including conventional cigarettes.[33]

TOBACCO CESSATION INTERVENTIONS

Treatment of adolescent tobacco use includes the use of pharmacotherapy as well as various psychosocial interventions. In guidelines put forth by the Department of Health and Human Services, all pediatric patients and their parents should be regularly screened for tobacco use by their health care providers and advised on abstinence with cessation advice and interventions.[34]

PHARMACOLOGIC INTERVENTIONS

Three classes of medications have been approved for smoking cessation: NRT (patch, gum, spray, inhaler, and lozenge), bupropion, and varenicline. These drugs have been shown in controlled clinical trials to be effective in adults, but data with adolescents are more limited with mixed results.

Nicotine Replacement Therapy

Several earlier trials looking specifically at the efficacy of NRTs in adolescents revealed safety, tolerability, and some promising efficacy with nicotine gum and transdermal patches. However, subsequent metaanalyses have suggested no significant effect of these pharmacotherapies for adolescent smokers,[35] with insufficient evidence to recommend any type of pharmaceutical treatment in young smokers.[36] A small trial with nicotine nasal spray also showed no efficacy among younger smokers and observed a large dropout rate from side effects.[37] More recent NRT trials with adolescents suggest that nicotine patch therapy appears to be greater when used with enhanced[38] versus more minimal[39] behavioral therapies, but long-term efficacy[40] is not supported. Although NRT is recognized as safe in adolescents,[38] smoking cessation medications are not Food and Drug Administration approved for use in those less than the age of 18. Nevertheless, national guidelines encourage NRT use in regular and not occasional adolescent smokers.[41] There is no evidence to support the use of e-cigarettes for smoking cessation among adolescents.

Bupropion

Bupropion SR is an antidepressant that exerts its effect primarily through the inhibition of dopamine reuptake and is also a weak noradrenaline reuptake inhibitor and an antagonist at postsynaptic nicotinic receptors. Only a small number of cessation trials to date, most enrolling older adolescents, have investigated bupropion SR.[42–45] Results are mixed, but suggest that use of this agent with psychosocial interventions can enhance cessation outcomes.

Varenicline

Varenicline is a partial agonist that binds to nicotinic receptors and reduces craving for nicotine. Clinical trials indicate that varenicline reduces relapse in abstinent smokers[46,47] and is more effective than bupropion in adults. A study on the pharmacokinetics, safety, and tolerability of varenicline in adolescent smokers[48] did not show continuous abstinence compared with placebo, but reduced smoking at follow-up for those receiving a higher dose and adverse events comparable to adults. A more recent larger multisite trial of varenicline did not show efficacy among youth.[49] Therefore, evidence to date does not support the use of varenicline for smoking cessation among adolescents.

BEHAVIORAL INTERVENTIONS

Given the mixed results with medications to treat adolescent nicotine dependence, counseling and behavioral interventions are highly recommended for adolescents.

Cognitive Behavioral Therapy

Cognitive behavioral therapy (CBT) is a structured, one-on-one intervention that has shown good efficacy in adolescents and can be delivered by trained professionals and paraprofessionals. This treatment is focused on problem solving, managing craving and negative moods, as well as identifying triggers and preventing relapse. For example, the American Lung Association's Not on Tobacco program, which teaches coping skills, has been thoroughly investigated and has shown efficacy.[50] CBT interventions have been shown to have better quit rates when compared with the use of brief information sessions among adolescents.[50,51] Furthermore, research indicates that the skills individuals learn through CBT remain after the completion of treatment.[52]

Motivational Therapies

Motivation-focused interventions are widely used for adolescent smoking cessation, although the empirical evidence for efficacy is mixed. These interventions are usually guided by motivational interviewing (MI),[53] an approach acknowledging and resolving ambivalence about behavior change, or the transtheoretical model,[54] whereby an individual moves through stages of motivation to quit. Data suggest MI is superior to self-help materials[55] and brief advice[56] in reducing the number of self-reported cigarettes per day. A review of the literature[57] indicates that motivational interventions can be delivered as an independent cessation intervention, but are best when combined with other behavioral interventions to engage and initiate adolescents in treatment before introducing a more intensive intervention.[57] For example, Project Ex, a high school–based cessation program that uses MI and other behavioral strategies in an interactive group format, has shown efficacy when compared with a control group.[58] Motivation to quit may be a mediator of tobacco cessation in adolescent users, and addressing motivational issues may lead to increased readiness to change.[59]

Contingency Management

Contingency management (CM) is a behavioral intervention based on the principles of operant conditioning, whereby adolescents are rewarded for achieving tobacco abstinence with money or other reinforcers. Low participation and retention rates in many adolescent trials suggest that adolescents typically do not find their substance use to be problematic and are particularly resistant to the concept of behavior change.[60] Behavioral interventions that use CM have been shown to be feasible and efficacious, with robust end-of-treatment abstinence rates.[61,62] Strategies, such as providing the intervention in a school setting, enhancing feasibility through the use of cotinine rather than CO levels to confirm abstinence, and combining CM with additional behavioral therapies have proven to be effective.

Community-based interventions, also known as Tobacco Free and Win or Quit and Win contests,[63] have shown some promise in reducing smoking. This program is initiated in a community setting to encourage everyone to refrain from tobacco products with a chance to win cash rewards in specified time intervals. In a review of Quit and Win programs, 8 of 11 demonstrated quit rates that were significantly higher than the typical quit rate of smokers making a quit attempt in the past year.[64] One youth study in Germany suggested a smoke-free class competition as a cost-effective way to encourage students to not initiate the use of tobacco products.[65]

NOVEL INTERVENTIONS

Novel experimental interventions for adolescent smokers have been gaining popularity in the literature and include smoking cessation interventions using telephone counseling,[66] text messaging,[67] peer mentoring,[68] and social media or virtual self-help interventions.[69] It is important to note that these interventions are often used in combination with other behavioral interventions, and that more evidence is needed to support their efficacy. In addition, mind-body interventions, such as mindfulness, yoga, hypnosis, and biofeedback,[70] have been illustrated as promising in the adult literature, but data supporting their efficacy in youth are limited. A 2016 review suggested that school-based yoga is a potentially efficacious strategy for improving adolescent health,[71] but this has not been extended as a tobacco intervention. Finally, a cognitive bias modification task, a variation of the alcohol Approach-Avoidance Task,[72] which has been investigated to see if the approach bias for cigarettes can be changed to improve the cessation rates in adolescents, has shown some promise.[73]

In summary, adolescent nicotine addiction is a serious health concern, especially in light of novel and enticing nicotine products, such as electronic cigarettes. There is some evidence to support efficacy of psychosocial interventions for cessation among adolescents, with elements of CBT and MI showing promise. In addition, the efficacy of pharmacologic treatments varies, depending on the age of the adolescent, as well as the severity of the nicotine use. Despite advances made in the treatment of nicotine use disorders in adolescents, many challenges persist. Interventions may need to be multimodal and tailored by addressing unique tobacco cessation needs of adolescents, including stage of change, gender, and culture. In addition, risks and benefits need to be addressed with each adolescent, depending on the product used and the available supporting data.

REFERENCES

1. Gentzke AS, Creamer M, Cullen KA, et al. Vital signs: tobacco product use among middle and high school students–United States, 2011-2018. MMWR Morb Mortal Wkly Rep 2019;68(6):157–64.
2. Gentzke AS, Wang B, Robinson JN, et al. Curiosity about and susceptibility toward hookah smoking among middle and high school students. Prev Chronic Dis 2019;16:E04.
3. Schroeder MJ, Hoffman AC. Electronic cigarettes and nicotine clinical pharmacology. Tob Control 2014;23(Suppl 2):ii30–5.
4. Miech R, Patrick ME, O'Malley PM, et al. What are kids vaping? Results from a national survey of US adolescents. Tob Control 2017;26(4):386–91.
5. Villanti AC, Johnson AL, Ambrose BK, et al. Flavored tobacco product use in youth and adults: findings from the first wave of the PATH study (2013-2014). Am J Prev Med 2017;53(2):139–51.
6. Hsu G, Sun JY, Zhu SH. Evolution of electronic cigarette brands from 2013-2014 to 2016-2017: analysis of brand websites. J Med Internet Res 2018;20(3):e80.
7. Corey CG, Ambrose BK, Apelberg BJ, et al. Flavored tobacco product use among middle and high school students–United States, 2014. MMWR Morb Mortal Wkly Rep 2015;64(38):1066–70.

8. Benowitz NL. Pharmacology of nicotine: addiction, smoking-induced disease, and therapeutics. Annu Rev Pharmacol Toxicol 2009;49:57–71.

9. Nestler EJ. Is there a common molecular pathway for addiction? Nat Neurosci 2005;8(11):1445–9.

10. DiFranza JR, Riggs N, Pentz MA. Time to re-examine old definitions of nicotine dependence. Nicotine Tob Res 2008;10(6):1109–11.

11. Doubeni CA, Reed G, Difranza JR. Early course of nicotine dependence in adolescent smokers. Pediatrics 2010;125(6):1127–33.

12. Chang CM, Edwards SH, Arab A, et al. Biomarkers of tobacco exposure: summary of an FDA-sponsored public workshop. Cancer Epidemiol Biomarkers Prev 2017;26(3):291–302.

13. SRNT Subcommittee on Biochemical Verification. Biochemical verification of tobacco use and cessation. Nicotine Tob Res 2002;4(2):149–59.

14. Prokhorov AV, Pallonen UE, Fava JL, et al. Measuring nicotine dependence among high-risk adolescent smokers. Addict behaviors 1996;21(1):117–27.

15. Wheeler KC, Fletcher KE, Wellman RJ, et al. Screening adolescents for nicotine dependence: the Hooked On Nicotine Checklist. J Adolesc Health 2004;35(3):225–30.

16. DiFranza JR, Wellman RJ, Ursprung WW, et al. The autonomy over smoking scale. Psychol Addict Behav 2009;23(4):656–65.

17. Wilens TE, Vitulano M, Upadhyaya H, et al. Concordance between cigarette smoking and the modified Fagerstrom Tolerance Questionnaire in controlled studies of ADHD. Am J Addict 2008;17(6):491–6.

18. Foulds J, Veldheer S, Yingst J, et al. Development of a questionnaire for assessing dependence on electronic cigarettes among a large sample of ex-smoking E-cigarette users. Nicotine Tob Res 2015;17(2):186–92.

19. Morean M, Krishnan-Sarin S, Sussman S, et al. Psychometric evaluation of the Patient-Reported Outcomes Measurement Information System (PROMIS) Nicotine Dependence Item Bank for use with electronic cigarettes. Nicotine Tob Res 2018. [Epub ahead of print].

20. Kandel DB, Schaffran C, Griesler PC, et al. Salivary cotinine concentration versus self-reported cigarette smoking: three patterns of inconsistency in adolescence. Nicotine Tob Res 2006;8(4):525–37.

21. Kentala J, Utriainen P, Pahkala K, et al. Verification of adolescent self-reported smoking. Addict behaviors 2004;29(2):405–11.

22. Slotkin TA. Nicotine and the adolescent brain: insights from an animal model. Neurotoxicol Teratol 2002;24(3):369–84.

23. Wiencke JK, Kelsey KT. Teen smoking, field cancerization, and a "critical period" hypothesis for lung cancer susceptibility. Environ Health Perspect 2002;110(6):555–8.

24. Ratajczak A, Feleszko W, Smith DM, et al. How close are we to definitively identifying the respiratory health effects of e-cigarettes? Expert Rev Respir Med 2018;12(7):549–56.

25. Hess CA, Olmedo P, Navas-Acien A, et al. E-cigarettes as a source of toxic and potentially carcinogenic metals. Environ Res 2017;152:221–5.

26. Tierney PA, Karpinski CD, Brown JE, et al. Flavour chemicals in electronic cigarette fluids. Tob Control 2016;25(e1):e10–5.

27. Kalman D, Morissette SB, George TP. Co-morbidity of smoking in patients with psychiatric and substance use disorders. Am J Addict 2005;14(2):106–23.

28. Dudas RB, Hans K, Barabas K. Anxiety, depression and smoking in schoolchildren–implications for smoking prevention. J R Soc Promotion Health 2005; 125(2):87–92.
29. Audrain-McGovern J, Leventhal AM, Strong DR. Chapter eight–the role of depression in the uptake and maintenance of cigarette smoking. In: De Biasi M, editor. International review of neurobiology, vol. 124. Amsterdam: Elsevier; 2015. p. 209–43.
30. van Amsterdam J, van der Velde B, Schulte M, et al. Causal factors of increased smoking in ADHD: a systematic review. Subst Use Misuse 2018;53(3):432–45.
31. Colton CW, Manderscheid RW. Congruencies in increased mortality rates, years of potential life lost, and causes of death among public mental health clients in eight states. Prev Chronic Dis 2006;3(2):A42.
32. McCabe SE, West BT, McCabe VV. Associations between early onset of E-cigarette use and cigarette smoking and other substance use among US adolescents: a national study. Nicotine Tob Res 2018;20(8):923–30.
33. Bold KW, Kong G, Camenga DR, et al. Trajectories of E-cigarette and conventional cigarette use among youth. Pediatrics 2018;141(1) [pii:e20171832].
34. King JL, Reboussin BA, Spangler J, et al. Tobacco product use and mental health status among young adults. Addict behaviors 2018;77:67–72.
35. Hammond CJ, Gray KM. Pharmacotherapy for substance use disorders in youths. J Child Adolesc Subst Abuse 2016;25(4):292–316.
36. Stanton A, Grimshaw G. Tobacco cessation interventions for young people. Cochrane Database Syst Rev 2013;(8):CD003289.
37. Rubinstein ML, Benowitz NL, Auerback GM, et al. A randomized trial of nicotine nasal spray in adolescent smokers. Pediatrics 2008;122(3):e595–600.
38. Moolchan ET, Robinson ML, Ernst M, et al. Safety and efficacy of the nicotine patch and gum for the treatment of adolescent tobacco addiction. Pediatrics 2005;115(4):e407–14.
39. Hurt RD, Croghan GA, Beede SD, et al. Nicotine patch therapy in 101 adolescent smokers: efficacy, withdrawal symptom relief, and carbon monoxide and plasma cotinine levels. Arch Pediatr Adolesc Med 2000;154(1):31–7.
40. Scherphof CS, van den Eijnden RJ, Engels RC, et al. Long-term efficacy of nicotine replacement therapy for smoking cessation in adolescents: a randomized controlled trial. Drug Alcohol Depend 2014;140:217–20.
41. Pbert L, Farber H, Horn K, et al. State-of-the-art office-based interventions to eliminate youth tobacco use: the past decade. Pediatrics 2015;135(4):734–47.
42. Gray KM, Carpenter MJ, Lewis AL, et al. Varenicline versus bupropion XL for smoking cessation in older adolescents: a randomized, double-blind pilot trial. Nicotine Tob Res 2012;14(2):234–9.
43. Killen JD, Robinson TN, Ammerman S, et al. Randomized clinical trial of the efficacy of bupropion combined with nicotine patch in the treatment of adolescent smokers. J Consult Clin Psychol 2004;72(4):729–35.
44. Muramoto ML, Leischow SJ, Sherrill D, et al. Randomized, double-blind, placebo-controlled trial of 2 dosages of sustained-release bupropion for adolescent smoking cessation. Arch Pediatr Adolesc Med 2007;161(11):1068–74.
45. Leischow SJ, Muramoto ML, Matthews E, et al. Adolescent smoking cessation with bupropion: the role of adherence. Nicotine Tob Res 2016;18(5):1202–5.
46. Gonzales D, Rennard SI, Nides M, et al. Varenicline, an alpha4beta2 nicotinic acetylcholine receptor partial agonist, vs sustained-release bupropion and placebo for smoking cessation: a randomized controlled trial. JAMA 2006;296(1): 47–55.

47. Tonstad S, Tonnesen P, Hajek P, et al. Effect of maintenance therapy with vareni-cline on smoking cessation: a randomized controlled trial. JAMA 2006;296(1): 64–71.

48. Faessel H, Ravva P, Williams K. Pharmacokinetics, safety, and tolerability of var-enicline in healthy adolescent smokers: a multicenter, randomized, double-blind, placebo-controlled, parallel-group study. Clin Ther 2009;31(1):177–89.

49. Gray KM, McClure E, Tomiko R, et al. Randomized controlled trial of varenicline for smoking cessation: main findings. Presented at Annual meeting of the Society for Research on Nicotine and Tobacco. In. San Francisco, CA, February 20-23, 2019.

50. Horn K, McGloin T, Dino G, et al. Quit and reduction rates for a pilot study of the American Indian Not On Tobacco (N-O-T) program. Prev Chronic Dis 2005; 2(4):A13.

51. Minary L, Cambon L, Martini H, et al. Efficacy of a smoking cessation program in a population of adolescent smokers in vocational schools: a public health evalu-ative controlled study. BMC Public Health 2013;13:149.

52. Laude JR, Bailey SR, Crew E, et al. Extended treatment for cigarette smoking cessation: a randomized control trial. Addiction 2017;112(8):1451–9.

53. Rollnick S, Miller WR. What is motivational interviewing? Behav Cogn Psychother 1995;23(4):325–34.

54. Prochaska JO, DiClemente CC. Stages and processes of self-change of smok-ing: toward an integrative model of change. J Consult Clin Psychol 1983;51(3): 390–5.

55. Dalum P, Paludan-Muller G, Engholm G, et al. A cluster randomised controlled trial of an adolescent smoking cessation intervention: short and long-term effects. Scand J Public Health 2012;40(2):167–76.

56. Audrain-McGovern J, Stevens S, Murray PJ, et al. The efficacy of motivational in-terviewing versus brief advice for adolescent smoking behavior change. Pediat-rics 2011;128(1):e101–11.

57. Barnett E, Sussman S, Smith C, et al. Motivational interviewing for adolescent substance use: a review of the literature. Addict behaviors 2012;37(12):1325–34.

58. Idrisov B, Sun P, Akhmadeeva L, et al. Immediate and six-month effects of Project EX Russia: a smoking cessation intervention pilot program. Addict behaviors 2013;38(8):2402–8.

59. McCuller WJ, Sussman S, Wapner M, et al. Motivation to quit as a mediator of to-bacco cessation among at-risk youth. Addict behaviors 2006;31(5):880–8.

60. Balch GI, Tworek C, Barker DC, et al. Opportunities for youth smoking cessation: findings from a national focus group study. Nicotine Tob Res 2004;6(1):9–17.

61. Cavallo DA, Cooney JL, Duhig AM, et al. Combining cognitive behavioral therapy with contingency management for smoking cessation in adolescent smokers: a preliminary comparison of two different CBT formats. Am J Addict 2007;16(6): 468–74.

62. Krishnan-Sarin S, Duhig AM, McKee SA, et al. Contingency management for smoking cessation in adolescent smokers. Exp Clin Psychopharmacol 2006; 14(3):306–10.

63. Cummings KM. Community-wide interventions for tobacco control. Nicotine Tob Res 1999;1(Suppl 1):S113–6.

64. O'Connor R, Fix B, Celestino P, et al. Financial incentives to promote smoking cessation: evidence from 11 quit and win contests. J Public Health Manag Pract 2006;12(1):44–51.

65. Hoeflmayr D, Hanewinkel R. Do school-based tobacco prevention programmes pay off? The cost-effectiveness of the 'Smoke-free Class Competition. Public Health 2008;122(1):34–41.
66. Heffner JL, Kealey KA, Marek PM, et al. Proactive telephone counseling for adolescent smokers: comparing regular smokers with infrequent and occasional smokers on treatment receptivity, engagement, and outcomes. Drug Alcohol Depend 2016;165:229–35.
67. Kong G, Ells DM, Camenga DR, et al. Text messaging-based smoking cessation intervention: a narrative review. Addict behaviors 2014;39(5):907–17.
68. Thomas RE, Lorenzetti DL, Spragins W. Systematic review of mentoring to prevent or reduce tobacco use by adolescents. Acad Pediatr 2013;13(4):300–7.
69. Brendryen H, Drozd F, Kraft P. A digital smoking cessation program delivered through internet and cell phone without nicotine replacement (happy ending): randomized controlled trial. J Med Internet Res 2008;10(5):e51.
70. Carim-Todd L, Mitchell SH, Oken BS. Mind-body practices: an alternative, drug-free treatment for smoking cessation? A systematic review of the literature. Drug and alcohol dependence 2013;132(3):399–410.
71. Khalsa SB, Butzer B. Yoga in school settings: a research review. Ann N Y Acad Sci 2016;1373(1):45–55.
72. Wiers RW, Eberl C, Rinck M, et al. Retraining automatic action tendencies changes alcoholic patients' approach bias for alcohol and improves treatment outcome. Psychol Sci 2011;22(4):490–7.
73. Kong G, Larsen H, Cavallo DA, et al. Re-training automatic action tendencies to approach cigarettes among adolescent smokers: a pilot study. Am J Drug Alcohol Abuse 2015;41(5):425–32.

Alcohol Use Disorders in Adolescents

Sarah M. Bagley, MD, MSc[a],*, Sharon Levy, MD, MPH[b],
Samantha F. Schoenberger, BA[a]

KEYWORDS

• Adolescents • Alcohol • Substance use • Binge drinking

KEY POINTS

• Alcohol remains the most commonly used substance among the adolescent (12–17 years old) age group.
• This article highlights developmental impacts of alcohol use, particularly exploring the epidemiology of binge drinking and polysubstance use.
• Specific consideration is given to differing rates of alcohol use between genders, individuals of diverse sexual identities, and races and ethnicities.
• The article concludes with recommendations for identifying and addressing teen alcohol use in the medical setting.

INTRODUCTION

Alcohol is the most commonly used substance during adolescence.[1] Alcohol use by adolescents has been in significant decline in the United States since the 1980s,[2,3] as part of a larger trend of increasing rates of abstinence from all substance use among high school–aged youth.[4] Despite this tremendous public health success, national surveys in 2018 reported a leveling off of alcohol use and a slight increase in binge drinking rates,[1] reinforcing the need for continued efforts to ensure continued progress.

According to the 2016 National Survey on Drug Use and Health (NSDUH), 9% of adolescents aged 12 to 17 years reported past-30-day alcohol use (the common definition of current drinkers) and 5% reported current binge drinking (>5 drinks in a 2-hour period). These rates have been decreasing since 2002 but still represent substantial alcohol use, and notably high-risk binge alcohol use, for this age group. Given the

Disclosure: The authors have no conflicts of interest or disclosures to declare. Dr S.M. Bagley is supported by an NIH Mentored Research Career Development Award (NIDA 1K23DA044324).
[a] Boston Medical Center, 801 Massachusetts Avenue, 2nd floor, Boston, MA 02118, USA;
[b] Division of Developmental Medicine, Boston Children's Hospital, 300 Longwood Avenue, Boston, MA 02115, USA
* Corresponding author.
E-mail address: sbagley@bu.edu

association between adolescent substance use and susceptibility to addiction in adulthood,[5,6] prevention and early intervention remain critical objectives.

Screening and brief intervention incorporated into medical care have proved to be a successful model for reducing risky alcohol use by adults,[7] and national guidelines recommend that routine medical care be used as an opportunity to identify and address teen drinking.[8] Addressing alcohol use among youth poses unique considerations and challenges for clinicians. Developmental, neurologic, and biopsychosocial differences between youth and adults require adaptations to prevention and intervention efforts for this age group. Tailored interventions that consider age and developmental context, gender, sexual identity, race, and the presence of chronic medical conditions have been recommended.

This article reviews known impacts of alcohol on the developing adolescent brain, demographic differences in adolescent alcohol use, co-use of alcohol with other substances, co-occurring mental health concerns, and binge drinking. It ends with recommendations for caring for teens that use alcohol.

THE ADOLESCENT BRAIN AND ALCOHOL

Adolescence is a developmental period characterized by rapid physical maturation, increased drive for independence, heightened saliency of social and peer interactions, and brisk brain development,[9] all of which are affected by genes, environment, and sexual hormones. The brain is especially susceptible to the effect of neurotoxins, including alcohol and other drugs, during this period of rapid growth.

During normal adolescent brain development, synaptic pruning (the elimination of underused neural pathways) results in decreased in gray matter, whereas myelination to support rapid and efficient signaling results in increases in white matter. Both of these processes are particularly vulnerable to the effects of alcohol.[6,10] The sophistication of the dopaminergic reward system that reinforces the effects of psychoactive substances such as alcohol contrasts with the immaturity of the prefrontal cortex's executive function hub. As a result, the dopamine neurotransmission and resulting pleasurable feeling that alcohol use enhances is not matched by consideration of the effects of use.[11] This imbalance drives adolescent behavior toward heavy alcohol consumption, which is the most common pattern of alcohol use by this age group. Ninety percent of underage alcohol consumption occurs within the context of binge drinking.[12]

Heavy alcohol use during adolescence is associated with both anatomic and neurophysiologic changes in the brain. Alcohol seems to increase the rate of gray matter pruning and also increases myelin deposition, ultimately resulting in greater white matter volume.[13] The implications of these changes are not completely understood, but it has been hypothesized that they may be maladaptive with alcohol causing harmful overpruning. In concordance with these neurophysiologic changes, prospective, long-term, longitudinal studies have established that alcohol use during adolescence is causally linked with lower educational attainment[14] and worsening verbal memory, visuospatial functioning, and psychomotor speed. The few studies that focus on girls suggest they are particularly susceptible to the effects of alcohol on white matter atrophy.[15,16] Future functional neuroimaging studies may provide much more detail, allowing a more robust understanding of the impacts of alcohol on brain development.

RISKS ASSOCIATED WITH ALCOHOL USE

Adolescents and adults alike experience harms associated with alcohol use, although adolescents are at heightened risk because of both the typical pattern of heavy, episodic drinking and the vulnerability of the developing brain. For adolescents, no level of alcohol consumption is considered safe or within a healthy range. Alcohol poisoning, alcohol-related motor vehicle crashes and other unintentional injuries,[17] sexual risk behaviors, dating violence, and sexual violence[18] are all associated with underage drinking. The Centers for Disease Control and Prevention (CDC) estimates an average of more than 4000 alcohol-related deaths of people less than 21 years of age occur each year in the United States,[19] and many more young people experience morbidity related to alcohol use. Alcohol use also interferes with self-care. Binge drinking disrupts sleep[20] and is associated with disordered eating.[21] For youth with chronic medical conditions such as diabetes or gastrointestinal disorders, drinking is associated with poorer medication adherence.[22]

Exposure to alcohol during adolescence is also associated with long-term harms. Earlier onset of use increases the risk for alcohol use disorder.[6] Binge drinking in 12th grade is one of the strongest predictors of alcohol use disorders in middle age.[23,24] Heavy drinking in adolescence is associated with premature death[25] and greater risk of early disability.[26] In addition, drinking during adolescence is associated with a higher risk of neurodegeneration, particularly in learning and memory centers in the brain,[27] which affects education attainment and memory.

RISK FACTORS FOR ALCOHOL USE DISORDER

It is estimated that 6.2% of US adults have an alcohol use disorder[28] and several risk factors are known to increase the likelihood of developing a problem. Age of alcohol initiation is one of the strongest predictive factors; individuals who start drinking before the age of 15 years are approximately 5 times more likely to develop an alcohol use disorder compared with those who initiate after age 18 years.[29] Alcohol use disorder also has a strong heritable component, with nearly 40% to 60% of the risk explained by genetic factors.[30] Environmental risk factors for alcohol use disorder include prenatal alcohol exposure, maternal depression, parental antisocial behavior, and experiencing maltreatment or neglect. Individual traits that increase the risk of developing an alcohol use disorder include childhood antisocial behavior, cognitive and learning, and attention disorders.[31,32] Hawkins and colleagues[31] and Marshall[32] offer succinct reviews of these factors.

EPIDEMIOLOGY OF ALCOHOL USE

Considerable differences in the rates of alcohol use between genders and individuals of different sexual identities, race, and ethnicity have all been described.

Gender

Although historically the prevalence of alcohol use has been much higher among boys and men, in recent years the gap has shrunk. In early adolescence to midadolescence, there is a higher incidence of girls who report drinking.[33,34] Girls who start to drink early (before age 15 years) progress to heavy drinking more quickly than boys. By late adolescence the trend reverses and there is a higher incidence and prevalence of alcohol use among young men. Gunn and Smith[35] (2010) postulated that disinhibition, depressed mood, and differences in family and peer relationships may explain gender differences in alcohol use.[35-37] Given that alcohol use among young women has increased over time,[38,39] gender differences are an important area of future research.

Sexual Identity

Sexual minority youth are at increased risk for alcohol use relative to their heterosexual peers,[40] and research into alcohol use by LGBTQ [Lesbian, Gay, Bisexual,

Transgender or Transsexual, Queer or Questioning]-identifying adolescents remains a public health issue priority.[41] Although the prevalence of lifetime alcohol use has been decreasing in recent years among heterosexual youth, this has not been true among LGBTQ youth. Boys who identify as gay have higher adjusted odds of lifetime use, early onset of use, past-30-day any use, and past-30-day heavy drinking compared with heterosexual boys. Girls who identify as lesbian have higher adjusted odds of early-onset use compared with heterosexual girls. These disparities remain true among bisexual boys and girls as well.[42]

Race

Rates of alcohol use are higher for white and Hispanic high school students (61.7% and 64.7% respectively) than African American students (51.3%).[38] Asian American youth have the lowest rates of alcohol consumption among the predominant ethnic groups in the United States.[43] However, national survey data significantly simplify demographic categories, thus obscuring differences within large ethnic groups.

Treatment accessibility and outcomes contrast significantly across adolescents of different races as well.[44,45] African American and Hispanic youth are less likely to receive substance use treatment compared with white adolescents,[45] and both black and Hispanic youth are less likely to complete treatment compared with white, Native American, and Asian-American youth[44] even when adjusting for income and insurance status. Religiosity is a protective factor and associated with lower rates of alcohol and other drug consumption, although the protective effects are strongest for white youth.[46]

Alcohol and Teen Pregnancy

Forty percent of high school seniors report having ever had sexual intercourse, and of the 30% of girls who reported having sex in the previous 3 months, 19% were impaired by alcohol or other drugs at the time.[38] Adolescents who have sex while impaired have high rates of unintended pregnancy[47]; more than 13% of pregnant adolescents less than 18 years of age report past-month alcohol use[47] compared with 7% of those aged 18 to 25 years. These findings highlight the importance of conversations about fetal alcohol effects, including fetal alcohol syndrome, particularly with young pregnant teens.[48]

CO-USE OF ALCOHOL AND OTHER SUBSTANCES
Marijuana

After alcohol, marijuana is the second most commonly used psychoactive substance used by adolescents. Lifetime alcohol users are more likely to report lifetime marijuana use compared with peers who do not drink.[4] Use of more than 1 substance is associated with truancy and use of illicit drugs besides marijuana. Concurrent use of alcohol and marijuana is reported by 20% of adolescents in national survey data.[49] High school seniors who report extreme binge drinking (>10 drinks) and those that use marijuana daily or more are at the highest risk.[49]

Tobacco and Other Nicotine Products

Alcohol and cigarette use during adolescence is highly correlated and associated with other drug use. In adolescents who report early initiation (before 16 years of age) of alcohol and cigarette use, the adjusted prevalence of daily cigarette use is 57%, daily/almost daily marijuana use is 19%, and ever taken a medication not prescribed is 40%. Among youth who have a susceptibility to e-cigarette use, the most commonly used tobacco product among youth, initiation of alcohol use is higher.[50–52]

Opioids

Seven out of 10 adolescents who report nonmedical use of prescription opioids combine these drugs with other substances. Fifteen percent report that they combine opioid use with alcohol usually or always,[53] substantially increasing the risk of overdose.[54] The mixture of codeine and alcohol, as known as purple drank, sizzurp, and lean, is an increasing public health concern among adolescents and young adults.[55] These substances are combined to amplify the relaxing, pleasant feeling that comes with use of either of the substances alone, and sometimes further mixed with energy drinks.[56] This combination increases the risk of overdose and long-term health consequences, such as liver and kidney damage.[57]

CO-OCCURRING MENTAL HEALTH AND ALCOHOL USE

A prior mental health disorder is associated with risk for first-time alcohol use as well as a transition from regular alcohol use to problematic use among adolescents.[58] Major depression is the psychiatric disorder that most commonly co-occurs with alcohol use disorder.[59] Wu and colleagues[60] (2010) found a significant association for girls between frequent or heavy drinking and anxiety disorders, although no association for boys was identified. In addition to a high prevalence of co-occurring alcohol use and mental health disorders, younger age of a first drink is associated with increased risk for suicidal ideation.[27,61]

BINGE DRINKING

Binge drinking is defined as the amount of alcohol consumption needed to reach a blood alcohol level of 0.08 g/dl within a 2-hour period. Because of differences in size and body composition, the definition of binge should be adjusted by age and sex as follows: 3 or more standard drinks over a 2-hour period for youth 9 to 13 years old, 4 or more drinks for boys and 3 or more drinks for girls aged 14 or 17 years, and 5 or more drinks for boys aged 16 years or older.[62] Studies that use the adult definition of binge drinking may under-report this behavior in adolescents.[63] Furthermore, adolescents often consume alcohol from alternative containers, making the reporting of a standard drink inaccurate, further increasing the risk of under-reporting binge drinking.

The 2017 Youth Behavior Risk Survey reports that 13.5% of students consumed at binge levels (using age-appropriate and sex-appropriate measures) on at least 1 day during the last 30 days.[38] Studies remain divided on gender and racial differences in binge drinking behavior, with some national surveys reporting highest rates among female youth (15.9% of white girls, 6.8% of black girls, and 16.0% of Hispanic girls)[38] and others reporting higher rates in boys compared with girls.[63] Binge drinking is a behavior that is often repeated. More than 60% of eighth graders and 62% of 10th graders who had engaged in binge drinking during the previous 2 weeks at the time of study participation stated that they did so on multiple occasions.[64]

IDENTIFYING AND ADDRESSING TEEN ALCOHOL USE IN MEDICAL SETTINGS

Approaching the topic of substance use with adolescents requires a developmentally friendly approach. Refraining from judgment and maintaining confidentiality when possible help to support a trusting relationship between patient and provider.

- Screening for alcohol use. The primary care setting provides an optimal space to have longitudinal conversations about substance use. Alcohol and other substance use can be quickly identified and preliminarily assessed using developmentally appropriate screening tools that can also help guide response and intervention. The Academy of Pediatrics and the Substance Abuse and Mental Health Services Administration recommend that screening, brief intervention, and referral to treatment be incorporated into routine medical adolescent care.[65] As outlined in the American Academy of Pediatrics clinical guideline, the following are validated brief screens and assessment guides.

- Screening tools. Health care professionals need brief, practical screening and assessment tools to accurately triage adolescents into previously identified actionable categories: from no past-year tobacco, drug, or alcohol use for whom positive reinforcement may sustain abstinence behavior/delay initiation of substance use[4]; to past-year tobacco, drug or alcohol use without associated problems for whom anticipatory guidance or brief medical advice may reduce use[4]; to patients who have substance use problems or disorders that could benefit from a brief intervention and/or a referral to treatment.[4] Although rates of screening for alcohol use in pediatric primary care seem to be increasing, suboptimal screening practices are common,[66] and inaccurate screening results in missed opportunities for intervention. Several brief screening tools for substance use have been validated for use with adolescents. These tools use 1 of 2 strategies: problem-based tools ask questions about problems related to substance use, whereas frequency-based tools rely on the number or pattern of past-year substance use to identify adolescents that are likely to meet criteria for a substance use disorder. The CRAFFT (Car, Relax, Alone, Forget, Family/friends, and Trouble) is an older, problem-based tool that is still commonly used.[67,68] Although popular in practice, the problem-based nature of the CRAFFT may encourage interview administration and concurrently discourage the recommended self-administration.[69] In addition, CRAFFT questions are not tied to a specific substance. As a result, CRAFFT results may suggest a substance use disorder but do not identify which substances are problematic. To address these issues, the National Institute for Alcohol Abuse and Alcoholism developed a 2-question frequency-based screen that can detect risk of an alcohol use disorder based on age and frequency of consumption.[70] More recently, new frequency-based tools that include questions on marijuana and nicotine have been developed and validated for use in pediatric primary care.[71,72] These brief new tools identify whether an adolescent has initiated substance use and also help determine the risk of having a substance use disorder with separate risk levels for alcohol, tobacco, and marijuana use.

BRIEF INTERVENTION

Brief intervention refers to a conversation between a patient and health care provider that is tailored to screen results, age and developmental status, personal characteristics, and individual strengths and is intended to prevent, delay, or decrease alcohol use. Clear, unambiguous messaging that nonuse is best for health has been recommended by the American Academy of Pediatrics,[65] the National Institute on Alcoholism and Alcohol Abuse,[8] and other governmental agencies and professional societies. Although the United States Preventive Services Task Force review found the knowledge base insufficient to determine the effectiveness of brief interventions for adolescent alcohol use, strategies that incorporate motivational strategies and include psychoeducation regarding alcohol and its impact on health have shown promise.[67,73,74] Several published guidelines give specific suggestions and examples of recommended brief intervention strategies for adolescents.[8,65]

- Referral to treatment. Adolescents who drink alcohol regularly, have had problems related to use, or who meet criteria for an alcohol use disorder could benefit from ongoing substance use counseling and support to reduce alcohol use, beyond a brief intervention. Several evidence-based therapies, including motivational interviewing,[75] cognitive behavior therapy,[76] contingency management,[77] and various family therapies can be delivered either individually or in a group setting. For most adolescents, effective treatment can consist of outpatient counseling with a primary care integrated behavioral health counselor or a behavioral health provider in the community that has experience in working with adolescents with substance use disorders. Intensive outpatient programs and partial hospital programs offer more intensive group and individual counseling that can help adolescents with severe substance use disorders achieve early sobriety before returning to full participation in the community. For some adolescents, particularly individuals with unstable co-occurring mental health disorders, polysubstance use, and those with unstable housing or at risk of homelessness, acute or long-term residential treatment may be beneficial. Alcohol withdrawal is rare among adolescents but requires medical intervention and support when it does occur. Individuals with a history of daily heavy alcohol use over a prolonged period should be evaluated for possible withdrawal symptoms and treated as appropriate. Although not approved for use in individuals less than 18 years of age, naltrexone is approved for adults and may be useful as part of a treatment plan for moderate to severe alcohol use disorder.
- Support for families. Parents can reduce the likelihood of early alcohol initiation. High-quality relationships between parents and children, parental modeling of healthy behaviors, monitoring, involvement in a child's daily life, limiting alcohol availability, and general communication have all been shown to delay alcohol initiation in adolescence.[78] Reduced levels of drinking during later adolescence can be predicted by some of these same strategies in addition to disapproval of drinking, and discipline.[78] Low-intensity parenting interventions, including computer-based delivery for 12 contact hours have been shown to decrease adolescent alcohol use, suggesting that small changes can affect the short-term trajectories and long-term effects of adolescent alcohol use.[79,80] Primary care providers can include anticipatory guidance regarding alcohol use early in a child's life by encouraging parents to be role models by using alcohol only in moderation and avoiding driving after drinking. By midchildhood, most children have been exposed to alcohol and parents can begin discussing their thoughts about alcohol use as well as introducing family alcohol policies. For adolescents with alcohol use disorders, parent-based interventions can support the benefits of adolescent treatment. Targeting parenting factors in adolescent drinking interventions mediates the effects on adolescent outcomes, with indirect effects on risk factors for substance use.[78,81,82] Parent-based interventions include general parenting practices, such as monitoring, supervision, and communication, and alcohol-specific parenting, such as limiting alcohol availability.[78,82]

SUMMARY

Alcohol use by adolescents is common and arguably one of the most important modifiable health risk behaviors for this age group because of the high burden of acute consequences and long-term impacts on the developing brain. Heavy, episodic drinking is the most common consumption pattern for youth, and heavy drinking escalates risks. Alcohol use frequently co-occurs with other substance use, and combination use increases the risk of overdose, particularly with opioids. Given the multiple significant impacts on development and health, physicians play an important role in identifying and addressing alcohol use. Universal screening consistently followed by targeted brief interventions designed to delay or decrease use are an important component of health care for this age group. Unambiguous messages that recommend nonuse as best for health and well-being are recommended, easy to deliver, and may have great impact on adolescent behavior.

REFERENCES

1. Johnston LD, Miech RA, O'Malley PM, et al. Monitoring the future: national survey results on drug use, 1975-2017: overview, key findings on adolescent drug use. Ann Arbor (MI): Inst Soc Res Univ Mich; 2018.
2. Substance Abuse and Mental Health Services Administration. Results from the 2015 national survey on drug Use and health: Detailed Tables. Rockville (MD): SAMHSA; 2016. Available at: https://www.samhsa.gov/data/sites/default/files/NSDUH-DetTabs-2015/NSDUH-DetTabs-2015/NSDUH-DetTabs-2015.htm#tab6-71b. Accessed January 16, 2017.
3. Johnston LD, O'Malley PM, Miech RA, et al. Monitoring the future national survey results on drug use, 1975-2015: overview, key findings on adolescent drug use. Ann Arbor (MI): Inst Soc Res Univ; 2016.
4. Levy S, Campbell MD, Shea CL, et al. Trends in abstaining from substance use in adolescents: 1975–2014. Pediatrics 2018;142(2):e20173498.
5. Grant BF, Dawson DA. Age at onset of alcohol use and its association with DSM-IV alcohol abuse and dependence: results from the National Longitudinal Alcohol Epidemiologic Survey. J Subst Abuse 1997;9:103–10.
6. Waller R, Murray L, Shaw DS, et al. Accelerated alcohol use across adolescence predicts early adult symptoms of alcohol use disorder via reward-related neural function. Psychol Med 2018;49(4):675–84.
7. Mertens JR, Chi FW, Weisner CM, et al. Physician versus non-physician delivery of alcohol screening, brief intervention and referral to treatment in adult primary care: the ADVISe cluster randomized controlled implementation trial. Addict Sci Clin Pract 2015;10:26.
8. National Institute on Alcohol Abuse and Alcoholism. Alcohol screening and brief intervention for youth: a practitioner's guide; pocket guide. 2011. Available at: http://pubs.niaaa.nih.gov/publications/Practitioner/YouthGuide/YouthGuidePocket.pdf. Accessed December 18, 2018.
9. Arain M, Haque M, Johal L, et al. Maturation of the adolescent brain. Neuropsychiatr Dis Treat 2013;9:449–61.
10. Gogtay N, Giedd JN, Lusk L, et al. Dynamic mapping of human cortical development during childhood through early adulthood. Proc Natl Acad Sci U S A 2004;101(21):8174–9.
11. Spear LP, Varlinskaya EI. Adolescence. Alcohol sensitivity, tolerance, and intake. Recent Dev Alcohol 2005;17:143–59.
12. Office of Juvenile Justice and Delinquency Prevention. Drinking in America: Myths, Realities, and Prevention Policy. Washington, DC: U.S. Department of Justice, Office of Justice Programs, Office of Juvenile Justice and Delinquency Prevention; 2005.
13. Squeglia LM, Gray KM. Alcohol and drug use and the developing brain. Curr Psychiatry Rep 2016;18(5):46.

14. Nguyen-Louie TT, Castro N, Matt GE, et al. Effects of emerging alcohol and marijuana use behaviors on adolescents' neuropsychological functioning over four years. J Stud Alcohol Drugs 2015;76(5):738–48.
15. Hommer D, Momenan R, Rawlings R, et al. Decreased corpus callosum size among alcoholic women. Arch Neurol 1996;53(4):359–63.
16. Agartz I, Shoaf S, Rawlings RR, et al. CSF monoamine metabolites and MRI brain volumes in alcohol dependence. Psychiatry Res 2003;122(1):21–35.
17. Hingson RW, Heeren T, Winter MR. Age at drinking onset and alcohol dependence: age at onset, duration, and severity. Arch Pediatr Adolesc Med 2006; 160(7):739–46.
18. Swahn MH, Bossarte RM, Sullivent EE. Age of alcohol use initiation, suicidal behavior, and peer and dating violence victimization and perpetration among high-risk, seventh-grade adolescents. Pediatrics 2008;121(2):297–305.
19. Centers for Disease Control and Prevention. Alcohol and public health: alcohol-related disease impact. Atlanta (GA): ARDI; 2016.
20. Popovici I, French MT. Binge drinking and sleep problems among young adults. Drug Alcohol Depend 2013;132(1–2):207–15.
21. Thompson-Memmer C, Glassman T, Diehr A. Drunkorexia: a new term and diagnostic criteria. J Am Coll Health 2018;1–7. https://doi.org/10.1080/07448481.2018.1500470.
22. Weitzman ER, Ziemnik RE, Huang Q, et al. Alcohol and marijuana use and treatment nonadherence among medically vulnerable youth. Pediatrics 2015;136(3):450–7.
23. Merline AC, O'Malley PM, Schulenberg JE, et al. Substance use among adults 35 years of age: prevalence, adulthood predictors, and impact of adolescent substance use. Am J Public Health 2004;94(1):96–102.
24. Patrick ME, Schulenberg JE. How trajectories of reasons for alcohol use relate to trajectories of binge drinking: National panel data spanning late adolescence to early adulthood. Dev Psychol 2011;47(2):311–7.
25. McCambridge J, McAlaney J, Rowe R. Adult consequences of late adolescent alcohol consumption: a systematic review of cohort studies. PLoS Med 2011; 8(2):e1000413.
26. Sidorchuk A, Hemmingsson T, Romelsjö A, et al. Alcohol use in adolescence and risk of disability pension: a 39 year follow-up of a population-based conscription survey. PLoS One 2012;7(8):e42083.
27. Zeigler DW, Wang CC, Yoast RA, et al. The neurocognitive effects of alcohol on adolescents and college students. Prev Med 2005;40(1):23–32.
28. Park-Lee E, Lipari RN, Hedden SL, et al. Receipt of services for substance use and mental health issues among adults: results from the 2016. RTI International based in Research Triangle Park (NC): National Survey on Drug Use and Health; 2017.
29. Dawson DA, Goldstein RB, Patricia Chou S, et al. Age at first drink and the first incidence of adult-onset DSM-IV alcohol use disorders. Alcohol Clin Exp Res 2008;32(12):2149–60.
30. Schuckit MA. Alcohol-use disorders. Lancet 2009;373(9662):492–501.
31. Hawkins JD, Catalano RF, Miller JY. Risk and protective factors for alcohol and other drug problems in adolescence and early adulthood: implications for substance abuse prevention. Psychol Bull 1992;112(1):64–105.
32. Marshall EJ. Adolescent alcohol use: risks and consequences. Alcohol Alcohol 2014;49(2):160–4.

33. Cheng HG, Anthony JC. A new era for drinking? Epidemiological evidence on adolescent male-female differences in drinking incidence in the United States and Europe. Soc Psychiatry Psychiatr Epidemiol 2017;52(1):117–26.

34. Cheng HG, Anthony JC. Male-female differences in the onset of heavy drinking episode soon after first full drink in contemporary United States: From early adolescence to young adulthood. Drug Alcohol Depend 2018;190:159–65.

35. Gunn RL, Smith GT. Risk factors for elementary school drinking: pubertal status, personality, and alcohol expectancies concurrently predict fifth grade alcohol consumption. Psychol Addict Behav 2010;24(4):617–27.

36. Loeber R, Stepp SD, Chung T, et al. Time-varying associations between conduct problems and alcohol use in adolescent girls: the moderating role of race. J Stud Alcohol Drugs 2010;71(4):544–53.

37. Bolland KA, Bolland JM, Tomek S, et al. Trajectories of adolescent alcohol use by gender and early initiation status. Youth Soc 2016;48(1):3–32.

38. Kann L. Youth risk behavior surveillance — United States, 2017. MMWR Surveill Summ 2018;67. https://doi.org/10.15585/mmwr.ss6708a1.

39. Johnston LD, O'Malley PM, Bachman JG, et al. Monitoring the future national results on adolescent drug use: overview of key findings. Ann Arbor (MI): Inst Soc Res Univ; 2013.

40. Ziyadeh NJ, Prokop LA, Fisher LB, et al. Sexual orientation, gender, and alcohol use in a cohort study of U.S. adolescent girls and boys. Drug Alcohol Depend 2007;87(2):119–30.

41. Marshal MP, Friedman MS, Stall R, et al. Sexual orientation and adolescent substance use: a meta-analysis and methodological review*. Addiction 2008;103(4): 546–56.

42. Fish JN, Baams L. Trends in alcohol-related disparities between heterosexual and sexual minority youth from 2007 to 2015: findings from the youth risk behavior survey. LGBT Health 2018;5(6):359–67.

43. Hahm HC, Lahiff M, Guterman NB. Acculturation and parental attachment in Asian-American adolescents' alcohol use. J Adolesc Health 2003;33(2):119–29.

44. Saloner B, Carson N, Cook BL. Explaining racial/ethnic differences in adolescent substance abuse treatment completion in the united states: a decomposition analysis. J Adolesc Health 2014;54(6):646–53.

45. Cummings JR, Wen H, Druss BG. Racial/ethnic differences in treatment for substance use disorders among U.S. adolescents. J Am Acad Child Adolesc Psychiatry 2011;50(12):1265–74.

46. Wallace JM, Delva J, O'Malley PM, et al. Race/ethnicity, religiosity and adolescent alcohol, cigarette and marijuana use. Soc Work Public Health 2007;23(2–3): 193–213.

47. Connery HS, Albright BB, Rodolico JM. Adolescent substance use and unplanned pregnancy: strategies for risk reduction. Obstet Gynecol Clin North Am 2014;41(2):191–203.

48. Allard-Hendren R. Alcohol use and adolescent pregnancy. MCN Am J Matern Child Nurs 2000;25(3):159–62.

49. Patrick ME, Veliz PT, Terry-McElrath YM. High-intensity and simultaneous alcohol and marijuana use among high school seniors in the United States. Subst Abuse 2017;38(4):498–503.

50. Nicksic NE, Barnes AJ. Is susceptibility to E-cigarettes among youth associated with tobacco and other substance use behaviors one year later? Results from the PATH study. Prev Med 2019;121:109–14.

51. McCabe SE, West BT, McCabe VV. Associations between early onset of e-cigarette use and cigarette smoking and other substance use among us adolescents: a national study. Nicotine Tob Res 2018;20(8):923–30.

52. Moss HB, Chen CM, Yi H. Early adolescent patterns of alcohol, cigarettes, and marijuana polysubstance use and young adult substance use outcomes in a nationally representative sample. Drug Alcohol Depend 2014;136:51–62.

53. Abuse NI on D. Teens mix prescription opioids with other substances 2013. Available at: https://www.drugabuse.gov/related-topics/trends-statistics/infographics/teens-mix-prescription-opioids-other-substances. Accessed December 19, 2018.

54. The Substance Abuse and Mental Health Services Administration is the publisher of the DAWN Report: Substance Abuse and Mental Health Services Administration, Center for Behavioral Health Statistics and Quality. (July 2, 2012). The DAWN Report: Highlights of the 2010 Drug Abuse Warning Network (DAWN) Findings on Drug-Related Emergency Department Visits. Rockville, MD.

55. Watkins M, MA MFT. Dangers of mixing alcohol and codeine. American Addiction Centers. Available at: https://americanaddictioncenters.org/codeine-addiction/dangers-of-mixing-with-alcohol. Accessed December 19, 2018.

56. Housman JM, Williams RD. Adolescent nonmedical use of opioids and alcohol mixed with energy drinks. Am J Health Behav 2018;42(5):65–73.

57. Publications | National Institute on Alcohol Abuse and Alcoholism | Harmful Interactions. Available at: https://pubs.niaaa.nih.gov/publications/Medicine/medicine.htm. Accessed December 19, 2018.

58. Conway KP, Swendsen J, Husky MM, et al. Association of lifetime mental disorders and subsequent alcohol and illicit drug use: results from the national comorbidity survey-adolescent supplement. J Am Acad Child Adolesc Psychiatry 2016; 55(4):280–8.

59. Schulte MT, Ramo D, Brown SA. Gender differences in factors influencing alcohol use and drinking progression among adolescents. Clin Psychol Rev 2009;29(6): 535–47.

60. Wu P, Goodwin RD, Fuller C, et al. The relationship between anxiety disorders and substance use among adolescents in the community: specificity and gender differences. J Youth Adolesc 2010;39(2):177–88.

61. Baiden P, Mengo C, Boateng GO, et al. Investigating the association between age at first alcohol use and suicidal ideation among high school students: evidence from the youth risk behavior surveillance system. J Affect Disord 2019; 242:60–7.

62. Donovan JE. Estimated blood alcohol concentrations for child and adolescent drinking and their implications for screening instruments. Pediatrics 2009; 123(6):e975–81.

63. Chung T, Creswell KG, Bachrach R, et al. Adolescent binge drinking. Alcohol Res 2018;39(1):5–15.

64. Patrick ME, Schulenberg JE. Alcohol use and heavy episodic drinking prevalence and predictors among national samples of american eighth-and tenth-grade students. J Stud Alcohol Drugs 2010;71(1):41–5.

65. Levy SJL, Williams JF, Committee on Substance Use and Prevention. Substance use screening, brief intervention, and referral to treatment. Pediatrics 2016; 138(1):e20161211.

66. Levy S, Ziemnik RE, Harris SK, et al. Screening adolescents for alcohol use: tracking practice trends of massachusetts pediatricians. J Addict Med 2017; 11(6):427–34.

67. Knight J, Shrier L, Bravender T, et al. A new brief screen for adolescent substance abuse. Arch Pediatr Adolesc Med 1999;153(6):591–6.
68. Knight JR, Sherritt L, Shrier LA, et al. Validity of the CRAFFT substance abuse screening test among adolescent clinic patients. Arch Pediatr Adolesc Med 2002;156(6):607–14.
69. Levy S, Knight JR. Screening, brief intervention, and referral to treatment for adolescents. J Addict Med 2008;2(4):215–21.
70. Levy S, Dedeoglu F, Gaffin JM, et al. A screening tool for assessing alcohol use risk among medically vulnerable youth. PLoS One 2016;11(5):e0156240. Vrana KE, ed.
71. Levy S, Weiss R, Sherritt L, et al. An electronic screen for triaging adolescent substance use by risk levels. JAMA Pediatr 2014;168(9):822–8.
72. Kelly SM, Gryczynski J, Mitchell SG, et al. Validity of brief screening instrument for adolescent tobacco, alcohol, and drug use. Pediatrics 2014;133(5):819–26.
73. Bernstein E, Bernstein J, Feldman J, et al. An evidence based alcohol screening, brief intervention and referral to treatment (SBIRT) curriculum for emergency department (ED) providers improves skills and utilization. Subst Abuse 2007;28(4):79–92.
74. Monti PM, Colby SM, Barnett NP, et al. Brief intervention for harm reduction with alcohol-positive older adolescents in a hospital emergency department. J Consult Clin Psychol 1999;67(6):989–94.
75. D'Amico EJ, Miles JNV, Stern SA, et al. Brief motivational interviewing for teens at risk of substance use consequences: a randomized pilot study in a primary care clinic. J Subst Abuse Treat 2008;35(1):53–61.
76. McHugh RK, Hearon BA, Otto MW. Cognitive behavioral therapy for substance use disorders. Psychiatr Clin North Am 2010;33(3):511–25.
77. Petry NM. Contingency management in addiction treatment | psychiatric times. Psychiatric Times 2002.
78. Ryan SM, Jorm AF, Lubman DI. Parenting factors associated with reduced adolescent alcohol use: a systematic review of longitudinal studies. Aust N Z J Psychiatry 2010;44(9):774–83.
79. Allen ML, Garcia-Huidobro D, Porta C, et al. Effective parenting interventions to reduce youth substance use: a systematic review. Pediatrics 2016;138(2). https://doi.org/10.1542/peds.2015-4425.
80. Yap MBH, Cheong TWK, Zaravinos-Tsakos F, et al. Modifiable parenting factors associated with adolescent alcohol misuse: a systematic review and meta-analysis of longitudinal studies. Addiction 2017;112(7):1142–62.
81. Sandler I, Schoenfelder E, Wolchik S, et al. Long-term impact of prevention programs to promote effective parenting: lasting effects but uncertain processes. Annu Rev Psychol 2011;62:299–329.
82. Bo A, Hai AH, Jaccard J. Parent-based interventions on adolescent alcohol use outcomes: a systematic review and meta-analysis. Drug Alcohol Depend 2018;191:98–109.

Cannabis Use and Consequences

Yasmin Mashhoon, PhD[a,b], Kelly A. Sagar, MA[a,c,d], Staci A. Gruber, PhD[a,c,d],*

KEYWORDS

- Cannabis • Marijuana • Adolescence • Recreational • Cognition • Neuroimaging
- Structure • Function

KEY POINTS

- National survey data have documented a decrease in the perception of risk and harm associated with cannabis use, which in past years has been associated with increased rates of use among adolescents and young adults.
- Age of cannabis use onset, particularly during early adolescence, can differentially influence the organization and function of brain regions that regulate cognitive processing.
- Detecting structural and cognitive alterations related to cannabis use in adolescence highlights the importance of ensuring early intervention and education to help prevent/limit recreational use in adolescents.

INTRODUCTION

The resurgent popularity of cannabis, frequently referred to as marijuana, is easily characterized by the sentiment "everything old is new again." References to the medical use of cannabis have been found in texts of numerous ancient cultures dating back thousands of years. The cannabis plant is composed of hundreds of chemical compounds, including Δ^9- tetrahydrocannabinol (THC), the primary psychoactive constituent prized by recreational consumers and cannabidiol (CBD), a primary nonintoxicating constituent of the plant touted for its potential therapeutic potential.[1] Although cannabis was added to the US Pharmacopeia in 1850, the Marijuana Tax Act of 1937 made the use of cannabis illegal, and in 1942 cannabis was removed from the

Disclosure Statement: The authors have nothing to disclose.
[a] Department of Psychiatry, Harvard Medical School, 2 West, Room 305, 401 Park Drive, Boston, MA 02215, USA; [b] Behavioral Psychopharmacology Research Laboratory, McLean Imaging Center, Mclean Hospital, 115 Mill Street, Mailstop 204, Belmont, MA 02478, USA; [c] Cognitive and Clinical Neuroimaging Core, McLean Hospital, McLean Imaging Center, 115 Mill Street, Mailstop 204, Belmont, MA 02478, USA; [d] Marijuana Investigations for Neuroscientific Discovery, McLean Hospital, McLean Imaging Center, 115 Mill Street, Mailstop 204, Belmont, MA 02478, USA
* Corresponding author. Mclean Hospital, 115 Mill Street, Mailstop 204, Belmont, MA 02478.
E-mail address: gruber@mclean.harvard.edu

pharmacopeia. In 1970 with the creation of the Controlled Substance Act, cannabis was classified as a Schedule 1 substance, defining it as having no currently accepted medical use, a lack of demonstrated safety, and a high abuse potential. Interest in the potential therapeutic properties of cannabis persisted, however, and in 1996, California became the first state to fully legalize medical cannabis (MC) use. To date, 33 states and Washington, DC, have fully legalized cannabis use for medical purposes, and 15 states have allowed limited MC products, specifically, those high in CBD. Among states that have legalized MC, 11 states and Washington, DC, have also approved recreational or adult cannabis use. Legal cannabis use is considered the fastest growing market in the United States; in 2017, spending on legal cannabis reached $8.5 billion in the United States and is projected to increase to $23.4 billion in 2022.[2]

Adolescence is a period marked by increased risk-taking behaviors, including experimentation with substance use, and the widespread legalization of cannabis/cannabis-derived products for medical and recreational purposes is likely to further influence patterns of cannabis use among adolescents. In fact, recent data from the Monitoring the Future survey[3,4] indicate that approximately 80% of high school seniors and 88% of young adults (18–30 years old) report cannabis is readily available and/or very easy to acquire.[3,4] Furthermore, 29% of high school seniors viewed regular cannabis use as harmful, compared with 44% of seniors surveyed just 5 years prior[3]; this finding is important because decreased perception of risk and harm dovetails with increased recreational use of cannabis among adolescents and young adults. Because critical maturational processes in brain structure and cognitive function occur during adolescence,[5–7] youth are particularly vulnerable to neural consequences associated with substance use. Furthermore, study findings suggest that the initiation of substance use during adolescence, relative to exposure during adulthood, increases the risk of neurocognitive decrements and developing substance use disorders.[8,9]

Cannabis constituents interact with the body's endogenous cannabinoid (eCB) system. The eCB consists of endogenous cannabinoids (endocannabinoids), enzymes that synthesize and degrade endocannabinoids, and cannabinoid receptors such as CB1, predominantly and widely distributed throughout the central nervous system, and CB2, distributed in both the central nervous system and the peripheral organs.[10,11] Importantly, increased endogenous eCB system activity has been shown to improve executive functioning, diminish behavioral stress reactivity, and increase natural reward signaling.[12–16] The eCB system is also significantly involved in regulating cellular homeostasis and neuroplasticity, refining structural connectivity between neurons, and contributing to neural growth.[12,17,18] These regulatory mechanisms are critical for normal brain maturational processes during adolescence. Because exogenous cannabinoids such as THC can impact the eCB system, early exposure to THC is likely to interfere with and disrupt neurodevelopmental processes.

CONSEQUENCES OF ADOLESCENT CANNABIS EXPOSURE
Cognition

Multiple cognitive domains are impacted by cannabis use, particularly among those who initiate use during adolescence. Several comprehensive reviews[19–23] have highlighted the impact of adolescent cannabis use on the brain, often focusing on neurocognitive function across a wide range of domains. A consensus of these reviews is that adolescent onset of cannabis use is associated with greater neurocognitive deficits compared with individuals who initiate cannabis use in adulthood.

Specifically, relationships have been observed between cannabis use and reduced performance on measures of spatial working memory, verbal and episodic memory, complex attention, and executive function (eg, decision making, planning, inhibitory control), with growing evidence to suggest deficits in processing speed. Significant associations have also been observed between cannabis use and increased attentional bias to cannabis cues,[24] as well as risky sexual behaviors and negative sexual health consequences.[25] In addition, longitudinal studies note that poorer inhibitory functioning in substance use-naïve adolescents aged 12 to 14 years is predictive of more frequent cannabis use when adolescents reached ages 17 to 18 years,[26] and the initiation of cannabis use early in adolescence is associated with poorer processing speed, attention, memory, and visuospatial functioning 3 years later.[27]

In contrast, 1 cross-sectional study reported no significant differences in inhibitory control between cannabis-using young adults and nonusing individuals,[28] and a recent review concluded that there are few clinically meaningful associations between cannabis use and cognitive functioning (eg, learning, delayed memory, processing speed, executive functioning, and attention) in adolescents and young adults.[29] It is possible that reported cognitive deficits may be related to residual effects from acute use or withdrawal, or that the magnitude and persistence of cognitive deficits in cannabis users may have been overstated in past studies.[29] To this end, although some studies have documented cognitive decrements that persist even after a month of monitored cannabis abstinence,[30] others have reported recovery of function after abstinence.[31–33] As such, it will be important to consider individual, or subpopulation, differences in susceptibility to cognitive decrements associated with cannabis use as the field evolves.

Findings from studies assessing overall intelligence in cannabis users have been relatively inconsistent. Although some studies have reported lower IQ among recreational cannabis users relative to nonusers, more recent longitudinal studies with larger sample sizes have contradicted these findings.[34,35] Notably, 1 longitudinal study that investigated twins discordant for cannabis use found that cannabis users demonstrated lower IQ scores compared with nonusers, but that cannabis-using twins did not demonstrate significantly lower IQ scores relative to their abstinent siblings,[34] suggesting that lower IQ scores could be related to other familial factors instead of a direct result of adolescent cannabis use.[34]

In addition, there are conflicting reports regarding the impact of cannabis on academic engagement. Some studies suggest that impaired functioning on measures of psychomotor speed, emotional control, learning, memory, and executive function is consistent with findings of lower grades, higher absenteeism, lower SAT scores, greater reported school difficulty, and decreased college degree attainment observed in cannabis-using adolescents and young adults.[36,37] Other studies challenge the specificity of cannabis as a causal factor in poor cognitive outcomes in young users, suggesting other risk liabilities, such as sociodemographics, other substance use, or familial factors may contribute to the complexity of functional and educational outcomes.[29,38]

Brain Structure

During adolescence and emerging adulthood, the brain undergoes significant experience-dependent gray matter (GM) synaptic pruning[39,40] and white matter (WM) myelination.[41] GM consists of neuronal cell bodies and regulates decision making and information processing, whereas WM consists of nerve axons that coordinate efficient communication among brain networks.[42] Neural refinements of GM and WM are critical for greater neural signaling efficiency, cognitive processing, and network connectivity.[43,44]

A significant body of literature has documented structural brain alterations within adolescent-onset cannabis users. Although findings are often bidirectional, several studies report alterations in GM cortical thickness and subcortical volumes in adolescents,[45] young adults,[46–48] and adults.[49,50] Furthermore, greater cerebellar volumes in adolescent cannabis users were shown to persist beyond 1 month of closely monitored abstinence.[51] Notably, some investigations have shown that altered structural morphology in adolescent cannabis users, such as smaller prefrontal cortex (PFC), orbitofrontal cortex, and parietal cortex and greater cerebellar volumes, are associated with increased cognitive dysfunction.[51–53] Furthermore, smaller hippocampal volume in adolescent cannabis users, relative to healthy non–cannabis-using counterparts, has been associated with poor performance on verbal learning and memory tests.[45] It is of note, however, that other studies have not reported significant differences in brain structure between cannabis users and comparison cohorts.[54,55]

CB1 receptors are primarily located on neurons, but they also exist on myelinating glial cells, thereby influencing changes in structural connectivity.[56] Accordingly, adolescent cannabis use may affect the normal trajectory of WM maturation. Abnormal structural findings[57] and decreases in WM integrity[58–63] have been observed in those who begin using cannabis during adolescence. More specifically, studies have reported decreased WM integrity in several PFC, limbic, parietal, and cerebellar tracts, which could reflect risk factors for psychological and cognitive dysfunction, as well as symptoms of cannabis use disorder in adolescent and emerging adult cannabis users.[58–60,62,64,65] Previous studies have documented decreased WM in cannabis users compared with nonusing controls subjects, which was primarily driven by lower WM fiber tract integrity measured in those with early onset cannabis use, defined as regular use before age 16. Interestingly, lower WM integrity in early onset users was inversely correlated with higher scores of impulsivity, although this relationship was not observed in those with who initiated cannabis use later (after age 16).[61] The unique relationship between decreased WM structural integrity and adverse behavioral consequences found in early-onset cannabis users highlights the importance of early intervention and education to help prevent or limit recreational cannabis use among adolescents.

Brain Function

Brain imaging techniques, including functional MRI, have facilitated the examination of the underlying neural substrates associated with cannabis use. Cannabis use is often associated with altered patterns of neural activation across multiple brain regions, although the direction and magnitude of findings seem to vary. Several reviews have summarized findings of altered brain activation in young cannabis users, which are typically noted in medial temporal and frontal cortices, as well as the cerebellum.[21–23]

Functional MRI studies designed to measure activation patterns in adolescent recreational cannabis users in particular have reported altered PFC, orbitofrontal, cingulate, parietal, insular, subcortical, limbic, and cerebellar activation during tasks testing implicit memory,[66] verbal working memory,[67,68] verbal learning,[69] spatial working memory,[70] attentional control,[71] reward processing,[72–74] affective processing,[75] and executive functioning.[76–79] Importantly, although young cannabis users frequently exhibit alterations in neural activity during task performance, the majority of studies report similar task performance in cannabis users and nonusers (as recently reviewed by Sagar and Gruber[20]). It is likely that cannabis users recruit additional brain regions to compensate for less efficient neural strategies to achieve comparable performance relative to nonusers.[19,80] Interestingly, although the majority of the literature has reported differences in brain function in those who use cannabis compared with those who do not, one longitudinal study did not detect significant differences between cannabis users and nonusers in frontoparietal network function.[81]

Collectively, many of the studies conducted to date report compelling evidence that regular exposure to cannabis during adolescence, a time period marking critical developmental changes in the brain, can disrupt healthy maturation of neural networks involved in higher-order cognitive functioning (**Box 1**). Although it is clear that cannabis may impact brain activity, several key variables likely moderate the effects of cannabis and may contribute to some of the heterogeneity across investigations.

MODERATING FACTORS INFLUENCING THE CONSEQUENCES OF CANNABIS USE

Overall, the studies highlighted suggest that adolescent onset of cannabis use is related to poorer cognitive function, altered functional activity, and structural changes

---

Box 1
Consequences of adolescent cannabis exposure

Cognition

- Relationships have been observed between cannabis use and decreased performance on measures of
  - Spatial working memory
  - Verbal and episodic memory
  - Complex attention
  - Executive function (eg, decision making, planning, inhibitory, control)
  - Processing speed

Brain structure

- A significant body of literature has documented structural brain alterations within adolescent onset cannabis users

- Although findings are often bidirectional, several studies have reported alterations in
  - regional brain volumes[45]
  - cortical thickness[46–48]
  - morphology[49,50]

- Alterations in brain structure have also been associated with poorer performance on cognitive tasks[51]

Brain function

- Cannabis use is often associated with altered patterns of neural activation across multiple brain regions, although the direction and magnitude of findings seem to vary

- Functional MRI studies designed to measure activation patterns in adolescent recreational cannabis users have reported altered PFC, orbitofrontal, cingulate, parietal, insular, subcortical/limbic, or cerebellar activation during tasks testing
  - Implicit memory[66]
  - Verbal working memory[67,68]
  - Verbal learning[69]
  - Spatial working memory[70]
  - Attentional control[71]
  - Reward processing[72–74]
  - Affective processing[75]
  - Executive functioning[76–79]

in the brain. Data also suggest increased frequency and magnitude (greater amounts of cannabis used) are related to greater neural alterations. Interestingly, increased cannabis use may be a trait characteristic of early-onset users. For example, Gruber and colleagues[82] found that those with early onset reported using twice as often and nearly 3 times as much cannabis per week relative to late-onset users, and subsequent studies indicate that earlier onset, greater frequency, and greater magnitude of use predict poorer executive functioning.[83] Accordingly, adults with early-onset cannabis use could have an additive vulnerability, given the susceptibility of the developing brain to cannabis combined with an increased likelihood of higher cannabis use relative to those with later onset. In addition, Filbey and colleagues[84] observed that, among early-onset users, the duration of cannabis use and greater magnitude of use were associated with increased cortical thickness of the right medial temporal lobe, whereas late-onset cannabis users exhibited thinner cortex measurements. Results suggest that increased cannabis use likely interferes with normal patterns of synaptic pruning, reflecting a departure from expected developmental processes.

Although frequency and magnitude are critical variables moderating the impact of cannabis use, few measures facilitate reliable quantification of the frequency or magnitude of use, or other important factors, including cannabis potency, product type, and route of administration. Historically, measurements of the magnitude, or amount, of cannabis consumed are often reported as joints, smokes per week, or puffs taken rather than quantifying the actual amount (eg, grams, milligrams) of cannabis consumed. In addition, assessments of frequency of cannabis use are often based on number of use episodes, irrespective of magnitude of cannabis consumed. Furthermore, there is a lack of consensus in defining chronic, regular, casual, or heavy cannabis use. These discrepancies have likely contributed significantly to inconsistent findings across studies. Recently developed tools like the Daily Sessions, Frequency, Age of Onset, and Quantity of Cannabis Use Inventory (DFAQ-CU)[85] are key for the standardization of cannabis use, which will further help to elucidate the impact of cannabis in various populations, thus informing public health initiatives, including educational and interventional strategies designed to limit recreational cannabis use during critical neuromaturational years.

In addition, recreational cannabis users often seek potent products (those with higher THC concentrations), to achieve greater effects. Interestingly, the average potency of recreational cannabis products has shifted from approximately 4% in 1995 to approximately 17% in 2017, reflecting an increase of over 300%.[86] Moreover, the United States has seen an increasing popularity of concentrates, which are novel products with THC levels often approaching 60% or more,[87] and modes of use like dabbing, in which the consumer receives a large bolus of a concentrate all at once. As exposure to higher THC levels has been associated with increased symptoms related to cannabis use disorder as well as a higher risk for cannabis use disorder,[88,89] psychosis,[90,91] and cognitive decrements,[92,93] future studies examining the impact of high potency products are clearly warranted.

Although THC may increase negative consequences, other nonintoxicating, potentially therapeutic cannabinoids, such as CBD, may be protective. Studies have shown that CBD can mitigate or decrease the negative effects often associated with increased THC exposure, including cognitive decrements,[94] neural alterations,[95] and adverse psychological experiences, such as psychotic-like symptoms and anxiety.[96,97] Unfortunately, levels of CBD have decreased as THC has increased in recreational cannabis,[86] leaving many traditional recreational products with low or undetectable levels of CBD. Taken together, harm reduction models focused on delaying the onset of cannabis use and potentially limiting THC exposure are important public policy considerations.

SUMMARY AND FUTURE DIRECTIONS

As the popularity of cannabis use continues to increase, research investigations must continue to explore the impact of cannabis use in adolescence. Overall, studies suggest that recreational cannabis use during adolescence is associated with alterations in cognitive performance and measures of brain structure and function. Further, additional studies have shown that adolescents and young adults who use cannabis may experience problems related to academic functioning. These findings are especially important given expanding access to novel modes of use and newly available high potency products, as well as the increasing number of MC patients.

Interestingly, the impact of cannabis use during adolescence may not extend to MC patients. In a recent longitudinal study of MC patients examined before the initiation of MC use and followed over the course of treatment, MC patients exhibited improved performance on tasks of executive function and potential normalization of brain activation patterns following 3 months of MC use.[98] Given that MC patients were generally middle-aged to older adults, findings further highlight age of onset as a critical moderating variable. In addition, because many patients used products with rich and varied cannabinoids, including products high in CBD, additional studies examining the impact of individual constituents on cognitive performance and other functional variables are important future steps.

Given evidence of negative cognitive and neural consequences associated with adolescent recreational cannabis use, policymakers should consider more rigorous age-related guidelines to reduce or limit adolescent exposure and prevent advertisers from directly targeting adolescents, who are among the most brand- and image-conscious consumers. Furthermore, policymakers should consider safe limits of cannabis use in terms of frequency, magnitude, mode of use, and product potency.

REFERENCES

1. Morales P, Hurst DP, Reggio PH. Molecular targets of the phytocannabinoids: a complex picture. Prog Chem Org Nat Prod 2017;103:103–31.
2. Arcview Market Research. The state of legal marijuana markets. 6th edition. Boulder (CO): Arcview Market Research and BDS Analytics; 2018.
3. Johnston LD, Miech RA, O'Malley PM, et al. Monitoring the Future national survey results on drug use, 1975-2017: overview, key findings on adolescent drug use. Ann Arbor (MI): Institute for Social Research, The University of Michigan; 2018.
4. Schulenberg JE, Johnston LD, O'Malley PM, et al. Monitoring the future national survey results on drug use, 1975-2016: volume II, college students and adults ages 19-55. Ann Arbor (MI): Institute for Social Research; 2017.
5. Eaton DK, Kann L, Kinchen S, et al. Youth risk behavior surveillance–United States, 2005. J Sch Health 2006;76(7):353–72.
6. Casey BJ, Giedd JN, Thomas KM. Structural and functional brain development and its relation to cognitive development. Biol Psychol 2000;54(1–3):241–57.
7. Casey BJ, Getz S, Galvan A. The adolescent brain. Dev Rev 2008;28(1):62–77.
8. Brown SA, Tapert SF. Adolescence and the trajectory of alcohol use: basic to clinical studies. Ann N Y Acad Sci 2004;1021:234–44.
9. Spear LP. Adolescent alcohol exposure: are there separable vulnerable periods within adolescence? Physiol Behav 2015;148:122–30.
10. Di Marzo V, Piscitelli F. The endocannabinoid system and its modulation by phytocannabinoids. Neurotherapeutics 2015;12(4):692–8.

11. Garcia-Arencibia M, Molina-Holgado E, Molina-Holgado F. Effect of endocanna-binoid signalling on cell fate: life, death, differentiation and proliferation of brain cells. Br J Pharmacol 2019;176(10):1361–9.

12. Egerton A, Allison C, Brett RR, et al. Cannabinoids and prefrontal cortical function: insights from preclinical studies. Neurosci Biobehav Rev 2006;30(5):680–95.

13. Filbey FM, DeWitt SJ. Cannabis cue-elicited craving and the reward neurocircuitry. Prog Neuropsychopharmacol Biol Psychiatry 2012;38(1):30–5.

14. Hill MN, McEwen BS. Involvement of the endocannabinoid system in the neurobehavioural effects of stress and glucocorticoids. Prog Neuropsychopharmacol Biol Psychiatry 2010;34(5):791–7.

15. Hill MN, Tasker JG. Endocannabinoid signaling, glucocorticoid-mediated negative feedback, and regulation of the hypothalamic-pituitary-adrenal axis. Neuroscience 2012;204:5–16.

16. Hurd YL, Michaelides M, Miller ML, et al. Trajectory of adolescent cannabis use on addiction vulnerability. Neuropharmacology 2014;76(Pt B):416–24.

17. Katona I, Freund TF. Multiple functions of endocannabinoid signaling in the brain. Annu Rev Neurosci 2012;35:529–58.

18. Diaz-Alonso J, Guzman M, Galve-Roperh I. Endocannabinoids via CB(1) receptors act as neurogenic niche cues during cortical development. Philos Trans R Soc Lond B Biol Sci 2012;367(1607):3229–41.

19. Sagar KA, Gruber SA. Marijuana matters: reviewing the impact of marijuana on cognition, brain structure and function, & exploring policy implications and barriers to research. Int Rev Psychiatry 2018;30(3):251–67.

20. Sagar KA, Gruber SA. Interactions between recreational cannabis use and cognitive function: lessons from functional magnetic resonance imaging. Ann N Y Acad Sci 2018;1451(1):42–70.

21. Lisdahl KM, Gilbart ER, Wright NE, et al. Dare to delay? The impacts of adolescent alcohol and marijuana use onset on cognition, brain structure, and function. Front Psychiatry 2013;4:53.

22. Batalla A, Bhattacharyya S, Yucel M, et al. Structural and functional imaging studies in chronic cannabis users: a systematic review of adolescent and adult findings. PLoS One 2013;8(2):e55821.

23. Jacobus J, Tapert SF. Effects of cannabis on the adolescent brain. Curr Pharm Des 2014;20(13):2186–93.

24. Cousijn J, Watson P, Koenders L, et al. Cannabis dependence, cognitive control and attentional bias for cannabis words. Addict Behav 2013;38(12):2825–32.

25. Schuster RM, Crane NA, Mermelstein R, et al. The influence of inhibitory control and episodic memory on the risky sexual behavior of young adult cannabis users. J Int Neuropsychol Soc 2012;18(5):827–33.

26. Squeglia LM, Jacobus J, Nguyen-Louie TT, et al. Inhibition during early adolescence predicts alcohol and marijuana use by late adolescence. Neuropsychology 2014;28(5):782–90.

27. Jacobus J, Squeglia LM, Infante MA, et al. Neuropsychological performance in adolescent marijuana users with co-occurring alcohol use: a three-year longitudinal study. Neuropsychology 2015;29(6):829–43.

28. Takagi M, Lubman DI, Cotton S, et al. Executive control among adolescent inhalant and cannabis users. Drug Alcohol Rev 2011;30(6):629–37.

29. Scott JC, Slomiak ST, Jones JD, et al. Association of Cannabis with cognitive functioning in adolescents and young adults: a systematic review and meta-analysis. JAMA Psychiatry 2018;75(6):585–95.

30. Medina KL, Hanson KL, Schweinsburg AD, et al. Neuropsychological functioning in adolescent marijuana users: subtle deficits detectable after a month of abstinence. J Int Neuropsychol Soc 2007;13(5):807–20.
31. Pope HG Jr, Gruber AJ, Hudson JI, et al. Neuropsychological performance in long-term cannabis users. Arch Gen Psychiatry 2001;58(10):909–15.
32. Fried PA, Watkinson B, Gray R. Neurocognitive consequences of marihuana–a comparison with pre-drug performance. Neurotoxicol Teratol 2005;27(2):231–9.
33. Hanson KL, Winward JL, Schweinsburg AD, et al. Longitudinal study of cognition among adolescent marijuana users over three weeks of abstinence. Addict Behav 2010;35(11):970–6.
34. Jackson NJ, Isen JD, Khoddam R, et al. Impact of adolescent marijuana use on intelligence: results from two longitudinal twin studies. Proc Natl Acad Sci U S A 2016;113(5):E500–8.
35. Mokrysz C, Landy R, Gage SH, et al. Are IQ and educational outcomes in teenagers related to their cannabis use? A prospective cohort study. J Psychopharmacol 2016;30(2):159–68.
36. Maggs JL, Staff J, Kloska DD, et al. Predicting young adult degree attainment by late adolescent marijuana use. J Adolesc Health 2015;57(2):205–11.
37. Meier MH, Hill ML, Small PJ, et al. Associations of adolescent cannabis use with academic performance and mental health: a longitudinal study of upper middle class youth. Drug Alcohol Depend 2015;156:207–12.
38. Verweij KJ, Huizink AC, Agrawal A, et al. Is the relationship between early-onset cannabis use and educational attainment causal or due to common liability? Drug Alcohol Depend 2013;133(2):580–6.
39. Huttenlocher PR. Synaptic density in human frontal cortex - developmental changes and effects of aging. Brain Res 1979;163(2):195–205.
40. Huttenlocher PR. Morphometric study of human cerebral cortex development. Neuropsychologia 1990;28(6):517–27.
41. Paus T, Zijdenbos A, Worsley K, et al. Structural maturation of neural pathways in children and adolescents: in vivo study. Science 1999;283(5409):1908–11.
42. Sporns O, Tononi G, Kotter R. The human connectome: a structural description of the human brain. PLoS Comput Biol 2005;1(4):e42.
43. Rakic P, Bourgeois JP, Goldman-Rakic PS. Synaptic development of the cerebral cortex: implications for learning, memory, and mental illness. Prog Brain Res 1994;102:227–43.
44. Dwyer JB, McQuown SC, Leslie FM. The dynamic effects of nicotine on the developing brain. Pharmacol Ther 2009;122(2):125–39.
45. Ashtari M, Avants B, Cyckowski L, et al. Medial temporal structures and memory functions in adolescents with heavy cannabis use. J Psychiatr Res 2011;45(8):1055–66.
46. Cousijn J, Wiers RW, Ridderinkhof KR, et al. Grey matter alterations associated with cannabis use: results of a VBM study in heavy cannabis users and healthy controls. Neuroimage 2012;59(4):3845–51.
47. Gilman JM, Kuster JK, Lee S, et al. Cannabis use is quantitatively associated with nucleus accumbens and amygdala abnormalities in young adult recreational users. J Neurosci 2014;34(16):5529–38.
48. Mashhoon Y, Sava S, Sneider JT, et al. Cortical thinness and volume differences associated with marijuana abuse in emerging adults. Drug Alcohol Depend 2015;155:275–83.
49. Matochik JA, Eldreth DA, Cadet JL, et al. Altered brain tissue composition in heavy marijuana users. Drug Alcohol Depend 2005;77(1):23–30.

50. Yucel M, Solowij N, Respondek C, et al. Regional brain abnormalities associated with long-term heavy cannabis use. Arch Gen Psychiatry 2008;65(6):694–701.

51. Medina KL, Nagel BJ, Tapert SF. Abnormal cerebellar morphometry in abstinent adolescent marijuana users. Psychiatry Res 2010;182(2):152–9.

52. Churchwell JC, Lopez-Larson M, Yurgelun-Todd DA. Altered frontal cortical volume and decision making in adolescent cannabis users. Front Psychol 2010; 1:225.

53. Price JS, McQueeny T, Shollenbarger S, et al. Effects of marijuana use on prefrontal and parietal volumes and cognition in emerging adults. Psychopharmacology (Berl) 2015;232(16):2939–50.

54. Block RI, O'Leary DS, Ehrhardt JC, et al. Effects of frequent marijuana use on brain tissue volume and composition. Neuroreport 2000;11(3):491–6.

55. Weiland BJ, Thayer RE, Depue BE, et al. Daily marijuana use is not associated with brain morphometric measures in adolescents or adults. J Neurosci 2015; 35(4):1505–12.

56. Moldrich G, Wenger T. Localization of the CB1 cannabinoid receptor in the rat brain. An immunohistochemical study. Peptides 2000;21(11):1735–42.

57. Medina KL, Nagel BJ, Park A, et al. Depressive symptoms in adolescents: associations with white matter volume and marijuana use. J Child Psychol Psychiatry 2007;48(6):592–600.

58. Arnone D, Barrick TR, Chengappa S, et al. Corpus callosum damage in heavy marijuana use: preliminary evidence from diffusion tensor tractography and tract-based spatial statistics. Neuroimage 2008;41(3):1067–74.

59. Ashtari M, Cervellione K, Cottone J, et al. Diffusion abnormalities in adolescents and young adults with a history of heavy cannabis use. J Psychiatr Res 2009; 43(3):189–204.

60. Bava S, Frank LR, McQueeny T, et al. Altered white matter microstructure in adolescent substance users. Psychiatry Res 2009;173(3):228–37.

61. Gruber SA, Dahlgren MK, Sagar KA, et al. Worth the wait: effects of age of onset of marijuana use on white matter and impulsivity. Psychopharmacology (Berl) 2014;231(8):1455–65.

62. Gruber SA, Silveri MM, Dahlgren MK, et al. Why so impulsive? White matter alterations are associated with impulsivity in chronic marijuana smokers. Exp Clin Psychopharmacol 2011;19(3):231–42.

63. Shollenbarger SG, Price J, Wieser J, et al. Poorer frontolimbic white matter integrity is associated with chronic cannabis use, FAAH genotype, and increased depressive and apathy symptoms in adolescents and young adults. Neuroimage Clin 2015;8:117–25.

64. Clark DB, Chung T, Thatcher DL, et al. Psychological dysregulation, white matter disorganization and substance use disorders in adolescence. Addiction 2012; 107(1):206–14.

65. Epstein KA, Kumra S. White matter fractional anisotropy over two time points in early onset schizophrenia and adolescent cannabis use disorder: a naturalistic diffusion tensor imaging study. Psychiatry Res 2015;232(1):34–41.

66. Ames SL, Grenard JL, Stacy AW, et al. Functional imaging of implicit marijuana associations during performance on an Implicit Association Test (IAT). Behav Brain Res 2013;256:494–502.

67. Jacobsen LK, Mencl WE, Westerveld M, et al. Impact of cannabis use on brain function in adolescents. Ann N Y Acad Sci 2004;1021:384–90.

68. Jacobsen LK, Pugh KR, Constable RT, et al. Functional correlates of verbal memory deficits emerging during nicotine withdrawal in abstinent adolescent cannabis users. Biol Psychiatry 2007;61(1):31–40.
69. Becker B, Wagner D, Gouzoulis-Mayfrank E, et al. The impact of early-onset cannabis use on functional brain correlates of working memory. Prog Neuropsychopharmacol Biol Psychiatry 2010;34(6):837–45.
70. Schweinsburg AD, Nagel BJ, Tapert SF. fMRI reveals alteration of spatial working memory networks across adolescence. J Int Neuropsychol Soc 2005;11(5): 631–44.
71. Abdullaev Y, Posner MI, Nunnally R, et al. Functional MRI evidence for inefficient attentional control in adolescent chronic cannabis abuse. Behav Brain Res 2010; 215(1):45–57.
72. Jager G, Block RI, Luijten M, et al. Tentative evidence for striatal hyperactivity in adolescent cannabis-using boys: a cross-sectional multicenter fMRI study. J Psychoactive Drugs 2013;45(2):156–67.
73. De Bellis MD, Wang L, Bergman SR, et al. Neural mechanisms of risky decision-making and reward response in adolescent onset cannabis use disorder. Drug Alcohol Depend 2013;133(1):134–45.
74. Chung T, Paulsen DJ, Geier CF, et al. Regional brain activation supporting cognitive control in the context of reward is associated with treated adolescents' marijuana problem severity at follow-up: a preliminary study. Dev Cogn Neurosci 2015;16:93–100.
75. Gruber SA, Rogowska J, Yurgelun-Todd DA. Altered affective response in marijuana smokers: an FMRI study. Drug Alcohol Depend 2009;105(1–2):139–53.
76. Behan B, Connolly CG, Datwani S, et al. Response inhibition and elevated parietal-cerebellar correlations in chronic adolescent cannabis users. Neuropharmacology 2014;84:131–7.
77. Cousijn J, Wiers RW, Ridderinkhof KR, et al. Individual differences in decision making and reward processing predict changes in cannabis use: a prospective functional magnetic resonance imaging study. Addict Biol 2013;18(6):1013–23.
78. Gruber SA, Dahlgren MK, Sagar KA, et al. Age of onset of marijuana use impacts inhibitory processing. Neurosci Lett 2012;511(2):89–94.
79. Tapert SF, Schweinsburg AD, Drummond SP, et al. Functional MRI of inhibitory processing in abstinent adolescent marijuana users. Psychopharmacology (Berl) 2007;194(2):173–83.
80. Kanayama G, Rogowska J, Pope HG, et al. Spatial working memory in heavy cannabis users: a functional magnetic resonance imaging study. Psychopharmacology (Berl) 2004;176(3–4):239–47.
81. Cousijn J, Vingerhoets WA, Koenders L, et al. Relationship between working-memory network function and substance use: a 3-year longitudinal fMRI study in heavy cannabis users and controls. Addict Biol 2014;19(2):282–93.
82. Gruber SA, Sagar KA, Dahlgren MK, et al. Age of onset of marijuana use and executive function. Psychol Addict Behav 2012;26(3):496–506.
83. Dahlgren MK, Sagar KA, Racine MT, et al. Marijuana use predicts cognitive performance on tasks of executive function. J Stud alcohol Drugs 2016;77:298–308.
84. Filbey FM, McQueeny T, DeWitt SJ, et al. Preliminary findings demonstrating latent effects of early adolescent marijuana use onset on cortical architecture. Dev Cogn Neurosci 2015;16:16–22.
85. Cuttler C, Spradlin A. Measuring cannabis consumption: psychometric properties of the daily sessions, frequency, age of onset, and quantity of cannabis use inventory (DFAQ-CU). PLoS One 2017;12(5):e0178194.

86. Chandra S, Radwan MM, Majumdar CG, et al. New trends in cannabis potency in USA and Europe during the last decade (2008-2017). Eur Arch Psychiatry Clin Neurosci 2019;269:5–15.

87. Smart R, Caulkins JP, Kilmer B, et al. Variation in cannabis potency and prices in a newly legal market: evidence from 30 million cannabis sales in Washington state. Addiction 2017;112(12):2167–77.

88. Freeman TP, Winstock AR. Examining the profile of high-potency cannabis and its association with severity of cannabis dependence. Psychol Med 2015;45(15):3181–9.

89. van der Pol P, Liebregts N, Brunt T, et al. Cross-sectional and prospective relation of cannabis potency, dosing and smoking behaviour with cannabis dependence: an ecological study. Addiction 2014;109(7):1101–9.

90. Di Forti M, Marconi A, Carra E, et al. Proportion of patients in south London with first-episode psychosis attributable to use of high potency cannabis: a case-control study. Lancet Psychiatry 2015;2(3):233–8.

91. Large M, Nielssen O. Daily use of high-potency cannabis is associated with an increased risk of admission and more intervention after first-episode psychosis. Evid Based Ment Health 2017;20(2):58.

92. Ramaekers JG, Kauert G, van Ruitenbeek P, et al. High-potency marijuana impairs executive function and inhibitory motor control. Neuropsychopharmacology 2006;31(10):2296–303.

93. Kowal MA, Hazekamp A, Colzato LS, et al. Cannabis and creativity: highly potent cannabis impairs divergent thinking in regular cannabis users. Psychopharmacology (Berl) 2015;232(6):1123–34.

94. Morgan CJ, Gardener C, Schafer G, et al. Sub-chronic impact of cannabinoids in street cannabis on cognition, psychotic-like symptoms and psychological well-being. Psychol Med 2012;42(2):391–400.

95. Yucel M, Lorenzetti V, Suo C, et al. Hippocampal harms, protection and recovery following regular cannabis use. Transl Psychiatry 2016;6:e710.

96. Bhattacharyya S, Morrison PD, Fusar-Poli P, et al. Opposite effects of delta-9-tetrahydrocannabinol and cannabidiol on human brain function and psychopathology. Neuropsychopharmacology 2010;35(3):764–74.

97. Zuardi AW, Shirakawa I, Finkelfarb E, et al. Action of cannabidiol on the anxiety and other effects produced by delta 9-THC in normal subjects. Psychopharmacology (Berl) 1982;76(3):245–50.

98. Gruber SA, Sagar KA, Dahlgren MK, et al. The grass might be greener: medical marijuana patients exhibit altered brain activity and improved executive function after 3 months of treatment. Front Pharmacol 2017;8:983.

Beyond the Bud
Emerging Methods of Cannabis Consumption for Youth

Cara A. Struble, MA[a,b], Jennifer D. Ellis, MA[a,b],
Leslie H. Lundahl, PhD[a,*]

KEYWORDS

- Cannabis • Δ-9-tetrahydrocannibinol • Concentrates • Edibles • Vaping • Youth
- Adolescence

KEY POINTS

- Adolescent cannabis use is extending to methods of concentrated Δ-9-tetrahydrocanni-binol (THC) consumption, including edibles, vaping, and dabbing.
- Use of concentrated THC is linked to serious negative consequences, including impaired executive function, inhibitory motor control, and psychosis.
- Little is known about both short- and long-term consequences of concentrated use during adolescence.

INTRODUCTION

Adolescent cannabis use has been linked to both short-term and long-term neurocognitive, academic, and health-related consequences.[1–4] Despite mounting evidence that cannabis use is particularly harmful during adolescence, youth in the United States increasingly perceive cannabis to be relatively low risk.[5,6] Recent advances in cultivation techniques have enabled the growth of new strains of cannabis plants with high concentrations of Δ-9-tetrahydrocannabinol (THC, the major psychoactive ingredient in cannabis).[7] In addition, high-potency THC can be extracted from plant material and reformulated as concentrates that are widely available in numerous forms including edibles, oils, and wax. Unfortunately, not much is known about the effects of these highly concentrated THC products, and empirical data on effects, characteristics, and consequences of these products when used during adolescence are limited.

Disclosure Statement: All authors declare no conflict of interest with respect to the conduct or content of this work.
^a Department of Psychiatry and Behavioral Neurosciences, Substance Abuse Research Division, Wayne State University, 3901 Chrysler Service Drive, Suite 2A, Detroit, MI 48201, USA;
^b Department of Psychology, Wayne State University, 5057 Woodward Avenue, 7th Floor, Detroit, MI 48202, USA
* Corresponding author.
E-mail address: llundahl@med.wayne.edu

Pediatr Clin N Am 66 (2019) 1087–1097
https://doi.org/10.1016/j.pcl.2019.08.012
pediatric.theclinics.com

In this article, the authors review trends in adolescent cannabis use and present a brief overview of the relationships among cannabis policy, attitude toward cannabis, and cannabis use. They also summarize relevant literature on high-potency THC along with emerging consumption techniques including ingestion (eg, edibles) and vaporization (eg, dab rigs and vape pens), along with their attendant risks. Finally, the authors discuss clinical applications and offer suggestions for future research on use of THC concentrates by adolescents.

TRENDS IN TEEN CANNABIS USE, PERCEPTIONS, AND ATTITUDES

Cannabis continues to be the most widely used illicit substance among adolescents.[5,6] Data from the 2018 Monitoring the Future (MTF) survey indicated approximately 11% of 8th graders, 28% of 10th graders, and 36% of 12th graders used cannabis in the last year.[6] The proportion of teens in grades 8, 10, and 12 reporting current daily or near-daily cannabis use is about 1%, 3%, and 6% respectively, with an even greater percentage (12% of 12th graders) indicating lifetime history of daily or near-daily cannabis use.[6] Gender differences in cannabis use seem to be narrowing in more recent years, although men continue to demonstrate higher rates of frequent cannabis use and cannabis vaping compared with women. Caucasian teens have the lowest levels of cannabis use during 8th grade, but these early racial and ethnic differences nearly disappear in later grades as Caucasian adolescents tend to exhibit higher cannabis use (traditional smoking and cannabis vaping) compared with African American and Hispanic teens. Cannabis use is suggested to be inversely related to socioeconomic status for adolescents, with higher estimates among those from lower socioeconomic households, although notably, cannabis vaping estimates are more similar across socioeconomic status.[6]

Cannabis has the lowest discontinuation rate of all substances in 12th graders. In 2018, only 18% of teens in the MTF survey who initiated cannabis use did not continue to use thereafter. This discontinuation rate is the lowest of any substance recorded by the survey in 22 years, suggesting that for teens, experimental cannabis use is giving way to consistent use.[6] In addition, when examining the degree and duration of highs attained by cannabis, the proportion of cannabis users who reported getting moderately to very high has been steady for over a decade at approximately 74%.[5,6] In terms of duration, 44% of cannabis users indicated staying high typically for 3 or more hours.[6] However, the typical duration of highs attained by cannabis has fluctuated in recent years, suggesting that more data are needed to draw conclusions on possible trends. For example, in 2017, 51% percent of adolescent cannabis users noted staying high for 3 or more hours at a time.[5] This is noteworthy because changes in duration of highs might be attributed to increased cannabis potency or greater use of THC concentrates.

As rates of adolescent cannabis use seem to be on an upswing, overall perceived risk associated with cannabis has been steadily declining since 2009.[5,6,8] For instance, just 27% of 12th graders believe that regular cannabis use carries great risk, whereas 12% report that experimental use poses a great risk.[6] Among 8th and 10th graders, the proportions believing that experimental use poses great risk are at the lowest levels ever recorded by the MTF survey (20% and 14%, respectively).[6] Factors that may be associated with reductions in perceived risks include changing social norms and cannabis legalization.[5] For the first time, most 12th graders are not in favor of prohibiting cannabis use in public areas, with just 48% against legalization of public cannabis use and 22% against legalization of private cannabis use. Conversely, 48% of 12th graders believe cannabis should be entirely legal.[6] With more states legalizing recreational cannabis use, there might be concomitant changes in both perceived and actual availability of cannabis, perceived risk of cannabis use, and rates of use. Although research has established a negative association between perceived risk and rates of use,[8] longitudinal studies are needed to establish a causal relationship between these factors.

EFFECTS OF LEGALIZATION ON AVAILABILITY, PERCEIVED RISK, AND USE

Cannabis policy has changed significantly over the past several years, with 10 states and the District of Columbia having legalized cannabis for recreational use for adults older than 21 years as of May 2019. Medical use is legal in 33 states and the District of Columbia. There has been a great deal of debate over whether permissive cannabis policies for adults lead to increases in youth cannabis use. For example, perceived risk of cannabis use decreased while cannabis use increased among 12th graders in California following decriminalization and among 8th and 10th graders in Washington following legalization of recreational use, but no differences were observed in Colorado following legalization of cannabis for recreational use.[8,9] The lack of change in Colorado could be attributed to the already low perceived risk and high rates of cannabis use among youth in this state before legalization of recreational cannabis use. A study using data from the National Survey on Drug Use and Health found a greater reduction in perceived risk and larger increases in cannabis abuse and dependence among adolescents aged 12 to 17 years following legalization of medical use in Colorado compared with trends observed in nonmedical cannabis states.[10] Although causation cannot be inferred from the aforementioned studies, these results suggest that permissive cannabis policies are associated with decreased perceived risk and increased adolescent cannabis use, although the results may somewhat depend on the state, age group, and the data source in question.

Given that dispensaries in states with legal medical and recreational cannabis often sell cannabis in highly potent forms (eg, edibles, vaping products, concentrates) that are less available in states without these permissive policies, it might be expected that cannabis-permissive states would also have higher rates of adolescent vaping and edible use. Although dispensaries are prohibited from selling cannabis products to adolescents, a study conducted in California indicated that approximately 25% of medical and nonmedical cannabis users sold products purchased at dispensaries to someone else in the past 90 days, suggesting that adolescents likely are able to obtain dispensary products illegally.[11] Consistent with findings from the adult literature,[12] among youth aged 14 to 18 years who use cannabis, about 68% of those in states with legal cannabis laws (ie, medical and recreational) report lifetime edible use and 51% report lifetime cannabis vaping. Conversely, among youth who use cannabis in states with no legal provisions, 52% report use of edibles and 36% report vaping. Further, longer duration of legal cannabis status and greater dispensary density are associated with higher likelihood of edible use and vaping among youth.[13] Finally, between 2013 and 2015, 91% of calls to US poison control centers following consumption of edible products occurred in states with decriminalized and legalized medical/recreational cannabis, and youth aged 13 to 19 years had the second highest number of calls.[14] The high number of poison control calls indicates that adolescents living in cannabis-permissive states may be more likely to acquire and use highly concentrated cannabis products such as edibles.

HIGH-POTENCY CANNABIS CONCENTRATES AND CONSUMPTION METHODS AMONG ADOLESCENTS

As a result of specialized cultivation techniques, the cannabis flower today is much more potent than a few decades ago.[6] Analysis of samples of cannabis seized by the US Drug Enforcement Administration reveal that potency has increased from approximately 4% THC in 1995 to 12% in 2014.[7] Further, as a result of legalization, concentrated THC products are available for purchase through dispensaries. Concentrated forms of THC are produced via solvent extraction of cannabinoids from the cannabis plant. Typically used solvents are butane or carbon dioxide.[15] Although these solvents are removed at the end of the extraction procedure, it is possible that residual traces remain and are ingested by the user.[16] The remaining concentrate can have more than 2 to 3 times the THC concentration of even the highest-potency cannabis flowers. For example, in Colorado, the Department of Revenue reported the average potency in concentrated products to be 68.6% THC, and some dispensary Websites advertise concentrate cartridges for vape pens containing more than 85% THC.[17,18] Emerging evidence suggests that cannabis products may not be accurately labeled; underestimating THC potency may lead to accidental overconsumption of THC.[19]

The use of such highly potent cannabis is concerning.[20] A growing literature is beginning to identify risks specific to high-potency cannabis, such as increased rates of cannabis use disorder among adults who use concentrates and impaired executive function and inhibitory motor control for those who smoke higher-potency cannabis.[18,21] Currently, very little is known about the consequences of highly potent THC use in adolescents, although it is very likely that youth, already vulnerable to long-term consequences associated with cannabis use, may be at particular risk for serious sequelae from use of high-potency cannabis.[22] One challenge in identifying potential risks is the array of products available, which includes liquids (eg, butane hash oil, distillate), soft solids (eg, wax, budder), and hard solids (eg, shatter, crumble).

EDIBLES

Edibles include drinks, food, and lozenges that have been infused with THC. Rates of edible use among adolescents are relatively high, particularly among those who already use cannabis. Studies suggest that 61% to 72% of adolescents who reported using cannabis also used edibles.[23,24] Edible consumption seems to be more popular among individuals who do not perceive edibles to be risky, as well as in states with legal cannabis.[11,12,24] A sample of youth in San Francisco, where medical cannabis has been legal since the 1990s, reported that they were able to obtain both homemade and dispensary-made edibles from other students.[25] Information about edibles is available from sites such as YouTube, which may not impose age restrictions on video viewing or discuss how to prevent overconsumption.[26]

The pharmacokinetic profile of edible cannabis differs from inhaled cannabis. For example, blood concentration of THC is significantly lower following oral ingestion relative to inhalation (eg, smoking and vaporizing), and the time to reach maximum THC concentration in the blood is significantly longer for edibles compared with smoked THC.[27] Although the effects of inhaled THC can be felt rapidly, plasma THC typically does not peak until 1 to 2 hours after oral ingestion of cannabis in most individuals. Similarly, one study found that heart rate was significantly elevated 30 minutes after smoking THC but not until 1.5 and 3 hours after ingesting an edible.[28] Heterogeneity exists, because some individuals do not reach this peak until 4 to 6 hours while others might show more than one peak.[29]

A defining feature of edibles is the unpredictable profile of effects, which is likely due to variable bioavailability, which ranges between 4% and 20% across studies. Bioavailability of THC seems to be influenced by several factors, including individual physiology and drug vehicle. Onset and duration of effects also can be influenced by the type of edible used, as THC absorbed through oral mucosa (eg, lozenges dissolved under the tongue) seems to have a more rapid onset than THC absorbed through the gut because it avoids first-pass metabolism by the liver.[30] Compared with smoking and vaporizing, edibles may produce a stronger effect among occasional users relative to regular users. For example, one study found that while both regular and occasional smokers described greater subjective effects after smoking or vaporizing cannabis compared with placebo, only occasional smokers rated greater subjective experiences after ingesting an edible relative to a placebo. Occasional smokers also demonstrated greater 11-hydroxy-THC concentrations in blood following ingestion, potentially contributing to their greater subjective ratings.[31]

Given variability in dosing accuracy on packaging, slow onset of effects, and relatively unpredictable effects of edible cannabis, it can be very difficult to determine appropriate doses; thus, it is relatively easy for individuals to accidently overconsume.[19,32] Adolescents seem to be at a particularly high risk of being hospitalized for cannabis overconsumption via ingestion. Short-term effects of edible cannabis overconsumption involve drowsiness, confusion, rapid heart rate, and irritability.[13] Overconsuming edibles can also be a frightening experience, which, in extreme cases, can involve more serious symptoms, such as short-term psychosis. A case series on 5 young adult (22–35 year old) daily cannabis smokers found that these individuals experienced new symptoms of short-term psychosis lasting 1 to 4 days after consuming 100 + mg THC edibles.[33] Although this is a very small sample, these reactions are particularly concerning because early use of cannabis has been associated with a greater likelihood of developing symptoms of psychosis in adulthood.[34] Researchers have yet to explore the link between edible use during adolescence and psychosis.

VAPORIZING TECHNIQUES

Vaporizing is becoming popular as technology advances and vaporizers become more widely available to the public. Vaporizing differs from traditional smoking in that it does not involve combustion and thus lacks the toxic biproducts of combustion (eg, benzene, toluene). This leads many to incorrectly assume that vaporizing is an unequivocally healthier alternative to smoking cannabis because it reduces exposure to potentially harmful carcinogens and toxic byproducts of cannabis smoke. Further, vaporizing cannabis might lead to fewer respiratory problems.[35] Methods of vaporizing cannabis include the use of specialized vape pens, dab rigs, and high-quality desktop vaporizers such as the Volcano Medic Vaporizer.[36]

According to the 2018 MTF survey, 12% of 10th graders and 13% of 12th graders vaped cannabis in the past year, a significant increase from the prior year. About 25% of adolescent cannabis users indicated vaping cannabis products at least once.[6] Because very little is known about which vaporizing methods are most common among adolescents (eg, dab rigs vs vape pens) and very little is known about the average THC potency of products being vaporized, it is difficult to accurately characterize potential consequences of vaping cannabis.

Vaporized THC and smoked THC seem to have similar pharmacokinetic profiles. After inhalation, THC is rapidly absorbed in the lungs, reaching peak plasma concentrations within 3 to 10 minutes.[27,29,37] One study found medical-grade vaporizers produced higher plasma concentrations at 30 and 60 minutes compared with smoked cannabis in active cannabis users, but there were no other differences over the 6-hour time course.[38] In a study of infrequent cannabis users, vaporized cannabis resulted in higher blood THC concentrations, greater subjective ratings of drug effect, dry mouth, and dry/irritated eyes following 10 mg and 25 mg THC, and higher ratings of paranoia at 25 mg THC, relative to the same doses of smoked cannabis. In addition, cognitive and psychomotor performances were more impaired after cannabis vaporization, with deficits persisting 6 to 8 hours postadministration.[39] These findings, in contrast to previous studies, suggest vaporized cannabis more efficiently delivers THC to the lungs. Bioavailability of inhaled THC ranges from 10% to 35%, depending on the inhalation device and puff topography (ie, volume, breath-holding interval, number, and duration of puffs),[37] and can be up to 55% with efficient medical grade vaporizers.[40]

A small number of studies have examined correlates of using vaporized cannabis products. One study of high school students found that using e-cigarettes to vaporize cannabis products was associated with being a man, younger, and a lifetime history of cannabis and e-cigarette use.[41] Similar results were found in a study of college students, which indicated that being a man and of a high socioeconomic status were associated with having vaporized cannabis. This study also found that greater openness to experience, greater approval of regular cannabis use, frequent nicotine vaping, and cannabis use were related to more frequent cannabis vaping.[42] These studies provide important information about characteristics of individuals who are likely to vaporize cannabis, and further research on adolescent samples is needed.

Vape Pens

Vape pens are discreet battery-powered devices that heat cannabis products to activate THC, which is then inhaled. Vape pens go by many different names, including e-cigs, juuls, e-hookahs, and mods. With increased commercial access to and use of vape pens for nicotine consumption, it is no surprise that teens find these devices appealing for use of cannabis concentrates. These devices are extremely versatile for cannabis users, with different modifications allowing users to vape dried flower, oils, and concentrated wax. For example, although the traditional dab rig requires use of a blow torch that might deter younger cannabis users, dabbing can be simplified with use of a modified vape pen known as a dab or wax pen. Youth seem to be using vape pens with high-potency concentrates, as students from a Connecticut high school reported using vape pens to vaporize hash oil and wax. Further, teens in this sample were 27 times more likely than adults to use a vape pen to vaporize cannabis.[42]

Among a national sample of adolescent cannabis users aged 14 to 18 years, 44% reported ever vaping cannabis with the majority (58%) most commonly using a vape pen. Concentrates were the products most typically vaped. Adolescents who preferred vaping to smoking revealed they considered vaping to be healthier, better tasting, more easily hidden from parents/teachers, and produced stronger effects compared with smoking.[23] Given these factors, vape pens might be associated with lower perceived risk of use, younger onset of and more frequent use, and increased risky behavior such as use of vape pens while driving.[43] Further, accumulating evidence suggests that vape pens are not as safe as believed. Cannabis oils typically used in vape pens are diluted with harmful additives such as propylene glycol and polyethylene glycol, which, when heated, produce acetaldehyde and formaldehyde.[44] At this time, long-term consequences of vaped cannabis are unknown.

Dabbing

"Dabbing" is a rather complicated method of vaporizing cannabis concentrates that requires many tools, including a dab rig (a modified water pipe created for oils and concentrates), a nail attached to the rig to heat the concentrate, a dabber to apply the dab of wax to the nail, a dome placed over the nail to contain the vaporized concentrate, and a blow torch to heat the nail. The user heats the nail with the blow torch until the desired temperature is reached, then uses the dabber to vaporize the concentrate. The vapor passes through the dab rig and is inhaled.

In adults, use of butane hash oil (BHO), a particularly potent concentrate, has been linked to increased tolerance and withdrawal symptoms, in addition to acute symptoms such as confusion, impaired memory, reality distortions, and losing consciousness.[45,46] In college students, more frequent BHO use is related to greater academic, occupational, and interpersonal difficulties, self-care problems, and risky behaviors.[47] Two case studies detailed 3 BHO users aged 17 to 34 years who developed severe psychotic symptoms resulting from BHO use.[48,49] Another case study described an 18-year-old woman hospitalized with severe pneumonitis with acute hypoxic respiratory failure as a result of dabbing.[50] Because the nail of a dab rig is typically heated until it is red, it can reach temperatures of 900 to 1075°F; inhalation of this vapor can potentially harm the lungs.[50,51] In addition to the clear risks associated with dabbing, the amateur production of BHO is worrisome. Production instructions and videos are available via the Internet and require relatively few resources. Butane, a flammable, volatile substance, has caused burns, explosions, and fires in improper BHO home production.[52] Further, analysis of 57 dab samples revealed that 80% were contaminated with residual solvents or pesticides that were then consumed during dabbing.[16,53]

RECOMMENDATIONS

Further development of prevention and intervention efforts for adolescent cannabis use is warranted. Programming that educates adolescents on the risks of high-potency cannabis use and emerging methods of consumption may be beneficial. Psychoeducation for parents might include information about changes in THC potency over time, especially for parents who might have used lower-potency cannabis during their teen years and do not consider use to be risky. Professionals should ensure that parents are knowledgeable about methods of use described in this article so that they can look for potential warning signs of use (eg, blow torch, empty cannabis oil cartridges, suspicious lozenges or drinks). As more states move toward legalizing cannabis for medical and/or recreational use, policy changes that specifically consider emerging methods of cannabis use may be vital in preventing cannabis-related problems among adolescents. For example, following several accidental edible overdoses, particularly among children and adolescents, some states passed laws requiring that cannabis products contain clear warnings on labels and limit the amount of THC in edible products.[54,55] Similar regulations on vaping and dabbing products may be necessary.

Medical professionals should learn to quickly recognize symptoms of cannabis overconsumption in adolescents. As discussed earlier, several acute symptoms have been associated with overconsumption of cannabis concentrates in youth and adults, including but not limited to drowsiness, confusion, rapid heart rate, irritability, panic, anxiety, nausea or vomiting, and short-term psychosis (eg, paranoia, delusions, hallucinations).[13,48,56] Professionals should attempt to get a detailed history of recent cannabis use, including quantity and frequency of use, products used, consumption method, and dosing. Keep in mind that even if products are labeled, the labels might not be accurate.[19]

Treatment of cannabis overconsumption depends on several factors (eg, age, clinical presentation, severity of symptoms). Unfortunately, there is no available antidote for cannabis overconsumption, and studies of pharmacologic intervention in adolescents are lacking. Thus, treatment should focus on reducing discomfort associated with overconsumption. Supportive therapy, which could involve placing the patient in a calm quiet room, might reduce some of the distress associated with panic and anxiety. Reminding the patient of the temporary nature of their discomfort may also be beneficial in reducing anxiety. Clearly, more research is needed on how best to manage cannabis overconsumption in adolescents.

FUTURE DIRECTIONS

This article highlights the dearth of research on the use of emerging forms of cannabis use among adolescents and the urgent need for future research in this area. Although demographic correlates of edible and vaporized cannabis use among adolescents have been identified, very little is known about co-occurring psychopathology among individuals who ingest or vaporize cannabis, which may be relevant to treatment. In addition, very little is known about short-term and long-term effects of use. In particular, it may be helpful for future studies to examine the effects of concentrates, relative to flower, on long-term development in adolescents. It may also be helpful for future studies to examine whether specific consequences, such as blackouts from cannabis use or memory problems, are associated with use of concentrates. Finally, developing a means of quantifying dose and concentration is necessary to continue this important area of research.

SUMMARY

Rates of THC concentrate use are high among adolescents who use cannabis, particularly in states with legal recreational and/or medical cannabis. Adolescents may perceive certain alternative consumption methods as preferable to smoking for several reasons, including stronger effects, the ability to use discreetly, and misperceptions that certain consumption methods (eg, vaping) are safer than smoking. Unfortunately, adolescents may be at particularly high risk of serious consequences associated with concentrate use, such as accidental overdose from edible cannabis. Medical professionals should be aware of the current trends in cannabis concentrate use in order to quickly identify and treat youth who present in medical settings following cannabis overconsumption.

REFERENCES

1. Meier MH, Hill ML, Small PJ, et al. Associations of adolescent cannabis use with academic performance and mental health: a longitudinal study of upper middle class youth. Drug Alcohol Depend 2015;156:207–12.
2. Jacobus J, Bava S, Cohen-Zion M, et al. Functional consequences of marijuana use in adolescents. Pharmacol Biochem Behav 2009;92:559–65.
3. Brook JS, Stimmel MA, Zhang C, et al. The association between earlier marijuana use and subsequent academic achievement and health problems: a longitudinal study. Am J Addict 2008;17:155–60.
4. Pedersen ER, Miles JN, Osilla KC, et al. The effects of mental health symptoms and marijuana expectancies on marijuana use and consequences among at-risk adolescents. J Drug Issues 2015;45:151–65.
5. Miech RA, Johnston LD, O'Malley PM, et al. Monitoring the future national survey results on drug use, 1975–2017: volume I, secondary school students. Ann Arbor (MI): Institute for Social Research, The University of Michigan; 2018.

6. Miech RA, Johnston LD, O'Malley PM, et al. Monitoring the future national survey results on drug Use, 1975–2018: volume I, secondary school students. Ann Arbor (MI): Institute for Social Research, The University of Michigan; 2019.

7. ElSohly MA, Mehmedic Z, Foster S, et al. Changes in cannabis potency over the last 2 decades (1995-2014): analysis of current data in the United States. Biol Psychiatry 2016;79(7):613–9.

8. Miech RA, Johnston L, O'Malley PM, et al. Trends in use of marijuana and attitudes toward marijuana among youth before and after decriminalization: the case of California 2007-2013. Int J Drug Policy 2015;26(4):336–44.

9. Cerdá M, Wall M, Feng T, et al. Association of state recreational marijuana laws with adolescent marijuana use. JAMA Pediatr 2017;171(2):142–9.

10. Schuermeyer J, Salomonsen-Sautel S, Price RK, et al. Temporal trends in marijuana attitudes, availability and use in Colorado compared to non-medical marijuana states: 2003-11. Drug Alcohol Depend 2014;140:145–55.

11. Lankenau SE, Fedorova EV, Reed M, et al. Marijuana practices and patterns of use among young adult medical marijuana patients and non-patient marijuana users. Drug Alcohol Depend 2017;170:181–8.

12. Borodovsky JT, Crosier BS, Lee DC, et al. Smoking, vaping, eating: Is legalization impacting the way people use cannabis? Int J Drug Policy 2016;36:141–7.

13. Borodovsky JT, Lee DC, Crosier BS, et al. U.S. cannabis legalization and use of vaping and edible products among youth. Drug Alcohol Depend 2017;177: 299–306.

14. Cao D, Srisuma S, Bronstein AC, et al. Characterization of edible marijuana product exposures reported to United States poison centers. Clin Toxicol 2016;54(9): 840–6.

15. Stockburger S. Forms of administration of cannabis and their efficacy. J Pain Manage 2016;9(4):381–6.

16. Raber JC, Elzinga S, Kaplan C. Understanding dabs: Contamination concerns of cannabis concentrates and cannabinoid transfer during the act of dabbing. J Toxicol Sci 2015;40(6):797–803.

17. Orens A, Light M, Lewandowski B, et al. Marijuana policy group. Market size and demand for marijuana in Colorado: 2017 market update. 2018. Available at: https://www.colorado.gov/pacific/sites/default/files/MED%20Demand%20and%20Market%20%20Study%20%20082018.pdf. Accessed June 10, 2019.

18. Glendale Green House. Oil and wax cartridges. 2019. Available at: https://www.glendalegreenhouse.com/oil-wax-cartridges/. Accessed June 10, 2019.

19. Vandrey R, Raber JC, Raber ME, et al. Cannabinoid dose and label accuracy in edible medical cannabis products. JAMA 2015;313(24):2491–3.

20. Resko S, Ellis JD, Early TJ, et al. Understanding public attitudes toward cannabis legalization: qualitative findings from a statewide survey. Subst Use Misuse 2019; 54(8):1247–59.

21. Ramaekers JG, Kauert G, van Ruitenbeek P, et al. High-potency marijuana impairs executive function and inhibitory motor control. Neuropsychopharmacology 2006;31(10):2296–303.

22. D'Amico EJ, Tucker JS, Pedersen ER, et al. Understanding rates of marijuana use and consequences among adolescents in a changing legal landscape. Curr Addict Rep 2017;4(4):343–9.

23. Knapp AA, Lee DC, Borodovsky JT, et al. Emerging trends in cannabis administration among adolescent cannabis users. J Adolesc Health 2019;64(4):487–93.

24. Friese B, Slater MD, Battle RS. Use of marijuana edibles by adolescents in California. J Prim Prev 2017;38(3):279–94.

25. Friese B, Slater MD, Annechino R, et al. Teen use of marijuana edibles: a focus group study of an emerging issue. J Prim Prev 2016;37(3):303–9.

26. Krauss MJ, Sowles SJ, Stelzer-Monahan HE, et al. "It takes longer, but when it hits you it hits you!": Videos about marijuana edibles on YouTube. Subst Use Misuse 2017;52(6):709–16.

27. Newmeyer MN, Swortwood MJ, Barnes AJ, et al. Free and glucuronide whole blood cannabinoids' pharmacokinetics after controlled smoked, vaporized, and oral cannabis administration in frequent and occasional cannabis users: identification of recent cannabis intake. Clin Chem 2016;62(12):1579–92.

28. Newmeyer MN, Swortwood MJ, Andersson M, et al. Cannabis edibles: blood and oral fluid cannabinoid pharmacokinetics and evaluation of oral fluid screening devices for predicting Δ9-tetrahydrocannabinol in blood and oral fluid following cannabis brownie administration. Clin Chem 2017;63(3):647–62.

29. Grotenhermen F. Pharmacokinetics and pharmacodynamics of cannabinoids. Clin Pharmacokinet 2003;42(4):327–60.

30. Huestis MA. Human cannabinoid pharmacokinetics. Chem Biodivers 2007;4(8): 1770–804.

31. Newmeyer MN, Swortwood MJ, Abulseoud OA, et al. Subjective and physiological effects, and expired carbon monoxide concentrations in frequent and occasional cannabis smokers following smoked, vaporized, and oral cannabis administration. Drug Alcohol Depend 2017;175:67–76.

32. Subritzky T, Pettigrew S, Lenton S. Issues in the implementation and evolution of the commercial recreational cannabis market in Colorado. Int J Drug Policy 2016; 27:1–12.

33. Hudak M, Severn D, Nordstrom K. Edible cannabis-induced psychosis: intoxication and beyond. Am J Psychiatry 2015;172(9):911–2.

34. Malone DT, Hill MN, Rubino T. Adolescent cannabis use and psychosis: epidemiology and neurodevelopmental models. Br J Pharmacol 2010;160(3):511–22.

35. Lee DC, Crosier BS, Borodovsky JT, et al. Online survey characterizing vaporizer use among cannabis users. Drug Alcohol Depend 2016;159:227–33.

36. Volcano Medic Vaporizer. PharmaSystems Inc. Available at: https://www.pharmasystems.com/index.php?route=product/product&product_id=3811. Accessed June 10, 2019.

37. Lucas CJ, Galettis P, Schneider J. The pharmacokinetics and the pharmacodynamics of cannabinoids. Br J Clin Pharmacol 2018;84(11):2477–82.

38. Abrams DI, Vizoso HP, Shade SB, et al. Vaporization as a smokeless cannabis delivery system: a pilot study. Clin Pharmacol Ther 2007;82(5):572–8.

39. Spindle TR, Cone EJ, Schlienz NJ, et al. Acute effects of smoked and vaporized cannabis in healthy adults who infrequently use cannabis: a crossover trial. JAMA Netw Open 2018;1(7):e184841.

40. Solowij N, Broyd SJ, van Hell HH, et al. A protocol for the delivery of cannabidiol (CBD) and combined CBD and Δ9-tetrahydrocannabinol (THC) by vaporisation. BMC Pharmacol Toxicol 2014;15:58–65.

41. Morean ME, Kong G, Camenga DR, et al. High school students' use of electronic cigarettes to vaporize cannabis. Pediatrics 2015;136(4):611–6.

42. Jones CB, Hill ML, Pardini DA, et al. Prevalence and correlates of vaping cannabis in a sample of young adults. Psychol Addict Behav 2016;30(8):915–21.

43. Budney AJ, Sargent JD, Lee DC. Vaping cannabis (marijuana): Parallel concerns to e-cigs? Addiction 2015;110(11):1699–704.

44. Troutt WD, DiDonato MD. Carbonyl compounds produced by vaporizing cannabis oil thinning agents. J Altern Complement Med 2017;23(11):879–84.

45. Loflin M, Earleywine M. A new method of cannabis ingestion: the dangers of dabs? Addict Behav 2014;39(10):1430–3.
46. Cavazos-Rehg PA, Sowles SJ, Krauss MJ, et al. A content analysis of tweets about high-potency marijuana. Drug Alcohol Depend 2016;166:100–8.
47. Meier MH. Associations between butane hash oil use and cannabis-related problems. Drug Alcohol Depend 2017;179:25–31.
48. Keller CJ, Chen EC, Brodsky K, et al. A case of butane hash oil (marijuana wax)-induced psychosis. Subst Abus 2016;37(3):384–6.
49. Pierre JM, Gandal M, Son M. Cannabis-induced psychosis associated with high potency "wax dabs". Schizophr Res 2016;172(1–3):211–2.
50. Anderson RP, Zechar K. Lung injury from inhaling butane hash oil mimics pneumonia. Respir Med Case Rep 2019;26:171–3.
51. Meehan-Atrash J, Luo W, Strongin RM. Toxicant formation in dabbing: the terpene story. ACS Omega 2017;2(9):6112–7.
52. Stogner JM, Miller BL. Assessing the dangers of "dabbing": Mere marijuana or harmful new trend? Pediatrics 2015;136(1). https://doi.org/10.1542/peds.2015-0454.
53. Alzghari SK, Fung V, Rickner SS, et al. To dab or not to dab: Rising concerns regarding the toxicity of cannabis concentrates. Cureus 2017;9(9):e1676.
54. Pardo B. Cannabis policy reforms in the Americas: a comparative analysis of Colorado, Washington, and Uruguay. Int J Drug Policy 2014;25(4):727–35.
55. Barrus DG, Capogrossi KL, Cates SC, et al. Tasty THC: promises and challenges of cannabis edibles. Research Triangle Park (NC): Methods Rep RTI Press; 2016. https://doi.org/10.3768/rtipress.2016.op.0035.1611.
56. Centers for Disease Control and Prevention. Marijuana and public health frequently asked questions. 2018. Available at: https://www.cdc.gov/marijuana/faqs/overdose-bad-reaction.html. Accessed June 10, 2019.

Prescription Opioid Misuse Among Adolescents

Jason A. Ford, PhD

KEYWORDS

- Adolescents • Prescription opioid misuse • Sociodemographic characteristics
- Social determinants • Sources and motives • Prevention, intervention, and treatment

KEY POINTS

- Drug overdose deaths are on the increase among adolescents and a significant portion of these deaths are attributable to prescription opioids.
- It is important to identify risk factors for prescription opioid misuse among adolescents related to sociodemographic characteristics, health-related factors, and social determinants.
- Characteristics of prescription opioid misuse, such as source and motive, help us to understand how misuse is associated with negative outcomes.
- It is important to identify how prescription opioid misuse during adolescence is associated with drug use and health-related problems in adulthood.
- The extant research must inform prevention and intervention strategies and approaches to treatment for prescription opioid misuse among adolescents.

BACKGROUND

The United States is in the midst of a major public health crisis associated with drug overdose deaths. Data from the US Centers for Disease Control and Prevention indicated that there were 70,237 drug overdose deaths in 2017.[1] This number is up nearly 100% from the 36,010 drug overdose deaths reported in 2007. Although most drug overdose deaths occur in adults over the age of 25, they are not uncommon in younger populations. Adolescents and young adults aged 15 to 24 accounted for nearly 8% of all overdose deaths in 2017 and the number of deaths in this age group has increased dramatically in recent years. In 2017, the overdose death rate (per 100,000) was 12.6 among adolescents and young adults, up from 3.7 in 2000.

The proliferation of drug overdose deaths is largely attributable to opioids; they accounted for roughly 68% of all overdose deaths in 2017. This includes 15,482

Disclosure Statement: There are no conflicts of interest to report.
Department of Sociology, University of Central Florida, Howard Phillips Hall, Orlando, FL 32816-1360, USA
E-mail address: Jason.Ford@ucf.edu

Pediatr Clin N Am 66 (2019) 1099–1108
https://doi.org/10.1016/j.pcl.2019.08.005
0031-3955/19/© 2019 Elsevier Inc. All rights reserved.

associated with heroin use, 14,495 associated with natural and semisynthetic opioids (eg, morphine, oxycodone, and hydrocodone), 3194 associated with methadone, and 28,466 associated with synthetic opioids other than methadone (eg, fentanyl, fentanyl analogs, and tramadol). Although recent spikes in drug overdose deaths are largely attributable to drugs such as heroin and fentanyl, nearly 25% of all drug overdoses in 2017 involved a prescription opioid.

The goal of this article is to summarize the scientific knowledge on prescription opioid misuse (POM) among adolescents in the United States. To do this, I rely heavily on data from the National Survey on Drug Use and Health (NSDUH), one of the leading epidemiologic surveys on drug use in the United States.[2] The NSDUH is representative of the noninstitutionalized population of the United States aged 12 and older. Several statistics throughput this article are from the 2017 NSDUH, the most recent data available, which includes 13,722 respondents aged 12 to 17 years. In addition to the NSDUH, this article highlights important findings from the extant literature on POM among adolescents.

PREVALENCE AND TRENDS
Prevalence

The 2017 NSDUH includes measures of both use and misuse of prescription drugs. Prescription opioid use (eg, hydrocodone, oxycodone, and tramadol products) is defined as the use of one's own prescription medication as directed by a doctor or the misuse of prescription drugs and is common among adolescents with 25.9% reporting lifetime use and 17.0% reporting use in the past year. The NSDUH defines POM as use in any way not directed by a doctor, including use without a prescription of one's own medication (nonmedical misuse); use in greater amounts, more often, longer than told to take the drug, or in any other way not directed by a doctor (medical misuse). POM is one of the most common forms of substance use among adolescents with 4.7% reporting lifetime misuse and 3.1% reporting misuse in the past year. It is also worth noting that heroin use is relatively uncommon among adolescents, because only 1.4% report lifetime use and 0.4% report use in the past year in the 2017 NSDUH.

Trends

The NSDUH data show that past year POM among adolescents decreased from 2002 to 2014: in 2002, 7.6% of adolescents reported past year POM, it decreased to 7.2% in 2006, to 6.3% in 2010, and 4.7% in 2014. Beginning in 2015 the NSDUH made a change to the prescription drug module, querying both use and misuse compared with nonmedical use, the term used before 2015. This change has made it difficult to compare trends. Since then, the prevalence of POM among adolescents has steadily decreased from 3.9% in 2015 to 3.5% in 2016 and 3.1% in 2017.

As a supplement to the NSDUH, I briefly discuss findings from the Monitoring the Future (MTF) Study, a school-based study of 8th-, 10th-, and 12th-grade students from public and private middle and high schools in the coterminous United States.[3] The MTF defines POM as the use of a drug (eg, acetaminophen with hydrocodone [Vicodin], oxycodone [OxyContin], and acetaminophen with oxycodone [Percocet]) not under the orders of a doctor. The most recent MTF is from 2018 and estimates that 3.4% of 12th graders report POM in the past year. With regard to trends in POM among 12th graders, prevalence was relatively stable from 2002 (9.4%) to 2009 (9.2%); since then POM has been on a steady decline, decreasing to 7.9% in

2012, 5.4% in 2015, and 3.4% in 2018. Trends in POM among adolescents seem to follow similar trends in the NSDUH and MTF, with the MTF showing slightly higher rates.

Prescribing

It is also useful to look at trends in prescribing, because research shows that trends in POM are correlated with trends in appropriate medical use of prescription opioids.[4] A study published in *Pain* showed that the number of opioid prescriptions among children and adolescents remained relatively stable from 1996 (2.2 million prescriptions) to 2012 (2.5 million prescriptions).[5] Importantly, this study found a significant increase in the rate of high opioid use, children or adolescents who received 5 or more opioid prescriptions. This study also found that opioid prescriptions for adults in general, and also family members of children and adolescents more than doubled between 1996 and 2012. This finding is significant, because a primary source of prescription opioids among adolescents is friends or relatives.[2]

SOCIODEMOGRAPHIC CHARACTERISTICS
Age

Data from the 2017 NSDUH show that the prevalence of POM increases with age, with 0.9% of 12-year-olds reporting misuse and 5.4% of 17-year-olds reporting misuse.

Sex

The prevalence of POM is slightly higher among girls (3.4%) compared with boys (2.7%) in the NSDUH. This finding may be attributed to gender differences in responses to strain or negative life events, because females seems to be more likely to respond with depression, which is highly correlated with POM.[6]

Race and Ethnicity

The prevalence of POM is lowest among Asians (1.8%), followed by whites (2.8%), blacks or African Americans (3.0%), Native Americans and Alaskan Natives (3.2%), those who identify more than 1 race (3.7%), Hispanics (3.8%), and lastly Native Hawaiian and other Pacific Islanders (4.0%). An article published in *Prevention Science* examined differences in correlates of POM between white, black or African American, and Hispanic adolescents in the NSDUH.[7] With numerous controls included in multivariable regression models, this study found no significant difference in POM among whites versus Hispanics or whites versus blacks. However, analytical models estimated separately identified unique correlates of POM between these racial/ethnic groups.

Geographic Residence

An article published in the *Journal of Rural Health* assessed rural/urban differences in POM among adolescents.[8] This study found that the risk of POM was slightly increased among adolescents who lived in rural or small urban areas compared with those who lived in large urban areas. The increased risk of POM among rural adolescents was associated with criminal activity, a low perceived risk associated with substance use, and greater use of emergency medical treatment.

Military

One area in need of further research is the impact of having a family member in the military. Data from the 2017 NSDUH indicate that the prevalence of POM is higher among adolescents who have a family member (ie, parents or siblings) in the military (4.7%) compared with those with no family members in the military (2.8%).

PHYSICAL AND MENTAL HEALTH
Overall Health

Data from the 2017 NSDUH indicate that overall health is associated with POM, because the prevalence of misuse is under 3% for adolescents who rate their health as excellent or very good, but nearly 14% of adolescents who report their overall health as poor report past year misuse.

Depression

Adolescents in the NSDUH who report a major depressive episode in the past year are more likely to report POM (6.7% vs 2.4%). A study published in *Drug and Alcohol Dependence* confirms the association between major depressive episode and opioid misuse, abuse, and dependence among adolescents.[9]

Disability Status

The NSDUH data indicate that POM is more common among adolescents with a disability (7.6% vs 3.6%). Further research is needed to better understand the increased risk of POM among adolescents with a disability.

Suicidal Ideation

The NSDUH does not ask adolescent respondents about suicidal ideation, but research has shown that POM increased the risk of suicidal ideation, making a plan for suicide, and attempting suicide among adolescents.[10]

Self-Control

There also seems to be a link between self-control and POM, with the risk for misuse being increased among those who are impulsive and have a preference for risky behavior.[11]

DELINQUENT BEHAVIOR AND VICTIMIZATION

Justice-involved populations are at increased risk for substance use. Research shows that POM increases the risk of both self-reported delinquency and arrest among adolescents while including several covariates in the analytical model.[12] Research also shows that victims of sexual assault[13] and child abuse[14] (emotional and physical, but not sexual) are at increased risk for POM.

Social Determinants

Family
Research shows that POM by a parent, especially the mother, increases the risk of POM during adolescence.[15] Research also shows that strong attachment to parents and high levels of monitoring or supervision are associated with decreased risk of POM.[16]

School
In a study of school status, POM was most common among adolescents who were not in school, followed by those in school but at risk for dropping out, then adolescents who were being home schooled, with adolescents who were in school and not at risk for dropping out with the lowest prevalence of misuse.[17] This study also showed that opioid use disorder symptoms were more likely to occur among adolescents who

were not in school and those in school but at risk for dropping out compared with those who were in school and not at risk for dropping out. Additional research shows that adolescents with a strong bond to school (eg, liked going to school, felt school work was meaningful, had teachers told them they were doing good work) were at decreased risk for POM.[18]

Peers
Risk of POM was increased when substance use was more common among peers and also when peers had attitudes that were more permissive of substance use.[19]

Religiosity
Adolescents with higher levels of religiosity (eg, church attendance and importance of religious beliefs) are at a decreased risk for substance use, including POM.[20]

Sports
Adolescents involved in sports are, in general, less likely to use drugs. However, a few studies identify a connection between involvement in contact sports during adolescence and POM.[21,22] The increased risk for POM may be due to the fact that athletes have greater access to opioids via both legal and diverted sources.

Neighborhood
Although most studies focus on individual-level predictors of POM, a few studies have examined neighborhood-level characteristics that increase risk for POM.[23] This research showed that adolescents who lived in neighborhoods with higher levels of social disorganization (eg, high crime, abandoned buildings, residential instability) and lower levels of social capital (eg, neighbors help one another, visit each other's home) were at increased risk for POM.

CHARACTERISTICS OF PRESCRIPTION OPIOID MISUSE

Characteristics of POM such as source and motive are important in identifying users who are at increased risk for negative outcomes. The literature suggests that people who obtain prescription opioids from more deviant sources (eg, steal or buy them) compared with more conventional sources (eg, from 1 doctor or free from friends or relatives),[24] and those who report recreational motives (eg, to get high or experiment) compared with self-treatment motives (eg, relieve physical pain or relax/relieve tension)[25] are at increased risk for more frequent POM, opioid use disorder, and the use of alcohol and other drugs.

Sources

According to data from the 2017 NSDUH, the most common sources of prescription opioids for misuse among adolescents include from a friend or relative for free (39.2%), from 1 doctor (26.0%), bought from a friend or relative (11.9%), took from a friend or relative without asking (7.3%), bought from a dealer or other stranger (6.6%), got some other way (4.8%), from more than 1 doctor (2.3%), and stole from a doctors' office, clinic, hospital, or pharmacy (1.9%).

Motives

Results from the 2017 NSDUH identify the most common motives among adolescents to be to relieve physical pain (41.6%), followed by to feel good or get high (21.7%), relax or relieve tension (10.7%), help with feelings or emotions (9.9%), experiment or see what it is like (8.8%), help with sleep (4.3%), increase or decrease the effects of other drugs (1.6%), some other reason (1.2%), and hooked or have to have the drug (0.04%).

LONG-TERM OUTCOMES
Substance Use Disorder Symptoms

In 2 separate studies, McCabe and colleagues[26] used data from the MTF to assess the association of POM during adolescence and substance use disorder symptoms in adulthood. Although the medical use of opioids did not increase risk, POM during adolescence increased the risk of various substance use disorder symptoms at age 35. Additionally, adolescents who reported motives related to pain relief, misused opioids with higher misuse potential, misused multiple prescription opioids, or reported medical use after POM were at increased risk for substance use disorder symptoms at age 35.[27]

Heroin

POM in childhood or early adolescence increases the risk of heroin use in young adulthood.[28,29] Specifically, adolescents who initiate POM before age 13 have the highest risk of transitioning to heroin use during young adulthood. A separate study found that an overwhelming majority of heroin users (77.3%) reported POM in their lifetime and that frequent POM (>40 times in their lifetime) increased risk for heroin use.[30] Finally, rates of heroin use among respondents who report POM increased dramatically between 2002 and 2014.[31]

Injection

Although there is little research on this topic among adolescents, it does seem that POM is associated with an increased risk of injection drug use, as well as human immunodeficiency virus or hepatitis C virus infection among young people.[32,33]

PREVENTION, INTERVENTION, AND TREATMENT

The extant research has identified factors that increase risk of POM and negative outcomes, as well as how POM in adolescence is associated with substance use during adulthood. This scientific knowledge must be the foundation of prevention and intervention strategies. To begin, given the increasing number of overdose deaths associated with opioids, medications that reverse opioid overdose such as naloxone should be more accessible to adolescents. In 2018, the US Surgeon General released an advisory stating that people who are likely to come into contact with individuals who use opioids should have access to and knowledge regarding the use of naloxone. Although first responders and emergency departments have access to naloxone, it should be more accessible for use in home and school settings.

Medical Education

It is critical to educate physicians and residents about opioid use and misuse among adolescents. An editorial appearing in *Substance Abuse*, the official publication of the Association for Medical Education and Research in Substance Abuse, calls for the following: a stronger focus on opioid misuse and appropriate prescribing during residency education, making greater use of existing resources on pain management and opioid misuse, and developing mentorship programs that emphasize pain management and addiction.[34]

Prevention Programs

Educational prevention programs targeting substance use among adolescents are ubiquitous. Unfortunately, these programs are dated and often do not include information specific to prescription drugs. This situation is problematic because most people perceive prescription drugs to be safer than traditional street drugs. Prevention programs must be adapted to include information on prescription drugs so that adolescents and their parents can be educated about risks, taught to safely use prescription medications (including information on proper storage and disposal), recognize overdose and know how to reverse the effects (using naloxone), and have access to treatment and recovery support.[35]

Research suggests that increasing knowledge associated with POM may not be enough to deter use. Rather, interventions should focus on the perception of risk (eg, understanding the seriousness of adverse effects) and risk aversion values (eg, the belief that pain relief is more important than the risks associated with opioids).[36] Finally, some research has been conducted on the effectiveness of Scenario-Tailored Opioid Messaging Program (STOMP) on parents who have children that have been prescribed opioids.[37] The STOMP intervention enhances perception of risk, increases opioid risk avoidance, and was related to better decision making associated with giving or withholding an opioid for pain management.

Medical Marijuana

There has been some discussion that increased access to marijuana may decrease some of the harmful effects of opioids. A study published in *Drug and Alcohol Dependence* used data from the MTF study to assess the relationship between medical marijuana laws and substance use among adolescents.[38] This study found that POM decreased among 8th graders but increased among 12th graders after a state enacted a medical marijuana law. Additional research highlights key differences in laws between states that seem to decrease the risk of POM.[39] The protective effect of medical marijuana laws seems to be decreased in states that have more stringent regulations (eg, fewer legal protections and no or limited access to dispensaries).

Medication-Assisted Treatment

Medication-assisted treatment (MAT) for opioid use disorders using medications such as buprenorphine, methadone, and naltrexone has been found to be effective when combined with other forms of treatment. This research shows that MAT is associated with decreased opioid use, a decreased risk for overdose deaths, less criminal offending, and a decreased risk of infectious disease transmission, as well as increasing social functioning and retention in treatment.[30] The majority of research on MAT focus on adult populations and more knowledge is needed regarding adolescents.[40] The existing research on adolescents shows that buprenorphine and naloxone prevents relapse,[41] is cost effective,[42] decreases craving, eliminates withdrawal symptoms, and is less stigmatized than methadone.[43] Importantly, the American Academy of Pediatrics released a policy statement advocating for increased access to MAT for opioid-addicted adolescents.[44]

SUMMARY

Data from epidemiologic surveys indicate a decrease in POM among adolescents in recent years. However, drug overdose deaths continue to increase, a significant number of these deaths are attributable to POM, and adolescents are not immune to this problem. The extant research has assessed factors that increase risk for

POM and negative outcomes, but continued research is needed to identify causal mechanisms. This scientific knowledge generated must be the foundation of prevention and intervention efforts and must identify which forms of treatment are most effective for adolescents with opioid use disorders.

REFERENCES

1. Hedegaard H, Miniño AM, Warner M. Drug overdose Deaths in the United States, 1999–2017. NCHS data Brief, no 329. Hyattsville (MD): National Center for Health Statistics; 2018.
2. Center for Behavioral Health Statistics and Quality. 2017 National Survey on Drug Use and Health: detailed tables. Rockville (MD): Substance Abuse and Mental Health Services Administration; 2018.
3. Miech RA, Johnston LD, O'Malley PM, et al. Monitoring the Future national survey results on drug use, 1975–2018: volume I, secondary school students. Ann Arbor (MI): Institute for Social Research, The University of Michigan; 2019.
4. McCabe SE, West BT, Veliz P, et al. Trends in medical and nonmedical use of prescription opioids among US adolescents: 1976-2015. Pediatrics 2017;139 [pii: e20162387].
5. Groenewald CB, Rabbitts JA, Gebert T, et al. Trends in opioid prescriptions among children and adolescents in the United States: a nationally representative study from 1996 to 2012. Pain 2016;157:1021–7.
6. Ford JA, Reckdenwald A, Marquardt B. Prescription drug misuse and gender. Subst Use Misuse 2014;49:842–51.
7. Ford JA, Rigg KK. Racial/Ethnic differences in factors that place adolescents at risk for prescription opioid misuse. Prev Sci 2015;16:633–41.
8. Monnat SM, Rigg KK. Examining rural/urban differences in prescription opioid misuse among US adolescents. J Rural Health 2016;32:204–18.
9. Edlund MJ, Forman-Hoffman VL, Winder CR, et al. Opioid abuse and depression in adolescents: results from the National Survey on Drug Use and Health. Drug Alcohol Depend 2015;152:131–8.
10. Baiden P, Graaf G, Zaami M, et al. Examining the association between prescription opioid misuse and suicidal behaviors among adolescent high school students in the United States. J Psychiatr Res 2019;112:44–51.
11. Ford JA, Blumenstein L. Self-Control and substance use among college students. J Drug Issues 2013;43:56–68.
12. Ford JA. Nonmedical prescription drug use and delinquency: an analysis with a national sample. J Drug Issues 2008;38:493–516.
13. Young A, Grey M, Boyd CJ, et al. Adolescent sexual assault and the medical and nonmedical use of prescription medication. J Addict Nurs 2011;11:25–31.
14. Austin AE, Shanahan ME, Zvara BJ. Association of child abuse and prescription opioid use in early adulthood. Addict Behav 2018;76:265–9.
15. Griesler PC, Hu M, Wall MM, et al. Nonmedical prescription opioid use by parents and adolescents in the US. Pediatrics 2019;143.
16. Donaldson CD, Nakawaki B, Crano WD. Variations in parental monitoring and predictions of adolescent prescription opioid and stimulant misuse. Addict Behav 2015;45:14–21.
17. Schepis TS, Teter CJ, McCabe SE. Prescription drug use, misuse, and related substance use disorder symptoms vary by educational status and attainment in U.S. adolescents and young adults. Drug Alcohol Depend 2018;189:172–7.

18. Ford JA. Non-medical prescription drug use among adolescents: the influence of bonds to family and school. Youth Soc 2009;40:336–52.

19. Ford JA. Social learning theory and non-medical prescription drug use among adolescents. Sociol Spectr 2008;28:299–316.

20. Ford JA, Hill TD. Religiosity and adolescent substance use: evidence from the National Survey on Drug Use and Health. Subst Use Misuse 2012;47:787–98.

21. Veliz PT, Boyd C, McCabe SE. Playing through pain: sports participation and nonmedical use of opioid medications among adolescents. Am J Public Health 2013;103:e28–30.

22. Veliz P, Boyd CJ, McCabe SE. Nonmedical use of prescription opioids and heroin use among adolescents involved in competitive sports. J Adolesc Health 2017; 60:346–9.

23. Ford JA, Sacra SA, Yohros A. Neighborhood characteristics and prescription drug misuse among adolescents: the importance of social disorganization and social capital. Int J Drug Policy 2017;46:47–53.

24. Schepis TS, Wilens TE, McCabe SE. Prescription drug misuse sources of controlled medications in adolescents. J Am Acad Child Adolesc Psychiatry 2019;58:670–80.

25. McCabe SE, Veliz P, Wilens TE, et al. Sources of nonmedical prescription drug misuse among US high school seniors: differences in motives and substance use behaviors. J Am Acad Child Adolesc Psychiatry 2019;58:681–91.

26. McCabe SE, Veliz P, Schulenberg JE. Adolescent context of exposure to prescription opioids and substance use disorder symptoms at age 35: a national longitudinal study. Pain 2016;157:2173–8.

27. McCabe SE, Veliz PT, Boyd CJ, et al. A prospective study of nonmedical use of prescription opioids during adolescence and subsequent substance use disorder symptoms in early midlife. Drug Alcohol Depend 2019;194:377–85.

28. Cerda M, Santaella J, Marshall BD, et al. Nonmedical prescription opioid use in childhood and early adolescence predicts transitions to heroin use in young adulthood: a national study. J Pediatr 2015;167:605–12.

29. Palamar JJ, Shearston JA, Dawson EW, et al. Nonmedical opioid use and heroin use in a nationally representative sample of US high school seniors. Drug Alcohol Depend 2016;158:132–8.

30. Mattick RP, Breen C, Kimber J, et al. Buprenorphine maintenance versus placebo or methadone maintenance for opioid dependence. Cochrane Database Syst Rev 2014;(2):CD002207.

31. Martins SS, Segura LE, Santaella-Tenorio J, et al. Prescription opioid use disorder and heroin use among 12-34 year-olds in the United States from 2002 to 2014. Addict Behav 2017;65:236–41.

32. Jordan AE, Blackburn NA, Des Jarlais DC, et al. Past-year prevalence of prescription opioid misuse among those 11 to 30 years of age in the United States: a systematic review and meta-analysis. J Subst Abuse Treat 2017;77:31–7.

33. Mars SG, Bourgois P, Karandinos G, et al. "Every 'never' I ever said came true": transitions from opioid pills to heroin injecting. Int J Drug Policy 2014;25:257–66.

34. Arora NS, Marcotte KM, Hopper JA. Reducing opioid misuse among adolescents through physician education. Subst Abus 2018;39:6–8.

35. Paltry E, Bratberg JP, Buchanan A, et al. Rx for addiction and medication safety: an evaluation of teen education for opioid misuse prevention. Res Social Adm Pharm 2019;15(8):917–24.

36. Voepel-Lewis T, Boyd CJ, McCabe SE, et al. Deliberative prescription opioid misuse among adolescents and emerging adults: opportunities for targeted interventions. J Adolesc Health 2018;63:594–600.

37. Voepel-Lewis T, Zikmund-Fisher BJ, Boyd CJ, et al. Effect of a scenario-tailored opioid messaging program on parents' risk perceptions and opioid decision-making. Clin J Pain 2018;34:497–504.

38. Cerda M, Sarvet AL, Wall M, et al. Medical marijuana laws and adolescent use of marijuana and other substances: alcohol, cigarettes, prescription drugs, and other illicit drugs. Drug Alcohol Depend 2018;183:62–8.

39. Powell D, Pacula RL, Jacobson M. Do medical marijuana laws reduce addictions and deaths related to pain killers? J Health Econ 2018;58:29–42.

40. Chang DC, Klimas J, Wood E, et al. Medication-assisted treatment for youth with opioid use disorder: current dilemmas and remaining questions. Am J Drug Alcohol Abuse 2018;44:143–6.

41. Marsh LA, Moore SK, Borodovsky JT, et al. A randomized controlled trial of buprenorphine taper duration among opioid-dependent adolescents and young adults. Addiction 2016;111:1406–15.

42. Polsky D, Glick HA, Yang J, et al. Cost-effectiveness of extended buprenorphine-naloxone treatment for opioid-dependent youth: data from a randomized trial. Addiction 2010;105:1616–24.

43. Moore SK, Guarino H, Marsh LA. "This is not who I want to be:" Experiences of opioid-dependent youth before, and during, combined buprenorphine and behavioral treatment. Subst Use Misuse 2014;49:303–14.

44. Ryan SA, Gonzalez PK, Patrick SW, et al. Medication-assisted treatment of adolescents with opioid use disorders. Pediatrics 2016;138 [pii:e20161893].

Prescription Stimulants
From Cognitive Enhancement to Misuse

Timothy E. Wilens, MD[a,b,*], Tamar Arit Kaminski, BS[c]

KEYWORDS

- Stimulant misuse • Nonmedical use of prescription stimulants
- Attention-deficit/hyperactivity disorder • ADHD • Transitional age youth
- College students

KEY POINTS

- Prescription stimulant misuse is associated with both short-term and long-term adverse outcomes.
- College students with fraternity affiliation, lower academic standing, and problematic substance use are at a higher risk for stimulant misuse.
- Recent studies examining the cognitive enhancing effects of prescription stimulants in healthy controls demonstrate stronger subjective relative to objective cognitive effects.
- Due to the correlates, impairments, and negative outcomes associated with stimulant misuse, providers are encouraged to closely monitor college students for stimulant misuse.

INTRODUCTION

Stimulant medications are among first-line agents in the treatment of attention-deficit/hyperactivity disorder (ADHD) across the life span. ADHD is prevalent in up to 9% of children,[1] with an estimated 8% of college students affected in the United States.[2] This neurobehavioral disorder is characterized by developmentally inappropriate levels of inattention, distraction, and/or hyperactivity and impulsivity. Although stimulants are considered safe and effective across age groups,[3] they are liable to misuse and diversion in adolescents and young adults, referred to in this article as transitional age youth (TAY) (for review, see Wilens and colleagues[4]). In this article, misuse is defined as using ADHD stimulants without a prescription or not following clinical

Disclosure: See last page of the article.
[a] Child & Adolescent Psychiatry, Massachusetts General Hospital, Boston, MA 02114, USA;
[b] Department of Psychiatry, Harvard Medical School, Boston, MA 02114, USA; [c] Pediatric Psychopharmacology Program, Division of Child Psychiatry, Massachusetts General Hospital, Boston, MA 02114, USA
* Corresponding author. Child Psychiatry Service, Massachusetts General Hospital, 55 Fruit Street, YAW 6A, Boston, MA 02114.
E-mail address: twilens@partners.org

guidelines when using a prescription (eg, nonmedical use). Misuse has increasingly been reported among TAY, particularly on college campuses, and has been associated with characteristics and behaviors distinct from other substance use.[5,6]

ATTENTION-DEFICIT/HYPERACTIVITY DISORDER

TAY are among the most vulnerable populations to the challenges that ADHD presents across academic, occupational, and interpersonal domains due to the increasing responsibility and independence associated with beginning work and college.[4] Managing and treating ADHD in this age group can be particularly difficult due to the emergence of comorbid psychopathologies, such as substance use disorder (SUD) and low rates of adherence to treatment.[4,7]

Although stimulant medications have a known potential for misuse, several recent, large studies have found a protective effect of therapeutic stimulant treatment of childhood ADHD on later SUD.[8,9] Ultimately, when treating TAY with ADHD with stimulants, it is necessary to carefully assess patients through psychiatric, addiction, social, cognitive, educational, medical, and family evaluations in order to mitigate increased liability for misuse at this age.[10]

PRESCRIPTION STIMULANT MISUSE AND DIVERSION
Prevalence and Sources

Stimulant misuse peaks in young adults, according to the "2017 National Survey on Drug Use and Health": 7.4% of young adults aged 18 years to 25 years reported past-year stimulant misuse compared with 1.8% of adolescents aged 12 years to 17 years and 1.7% of adults aged 26 and above.[11] Past-year prescription stimulant misuse in young adults has eclipsed past-year use of opioids as the most prevalent prescription misused.[11] The substantial rate of stimulant misuse among young adults is concerning due to the impairments, correlates, and associated perceptions.

The most common source of stimulants for adolescents[12] and young adults[13] has been consistently found to be peers, and, in accordance, a substantial proportion of individuals have been found to divert (sell, trade, or give away) their medication in high school[14] and college.[15] Furthermore, diversion has been found to be associated with misusing a prescription as well as using other substances in both age groups.[16,17]

Demographic Characteristics of Stimulant Misusers and High-Risk Groups

Certain demographic characteristics have been found associated with higher risk of stimulant misuse. For example, a higher incidence of misuse among whites and men has been reported.[18] The literature is inconsistent in regard to gender differences in motivations for and severity of stimulant misuse. Some studies have reported that women were more likely than men to use stimulants to lose weight[19] and may be at greater risk to develop dependence than male users.[20] Also, available demographic data on stimulant misuse are based on studies of college students due to the high prevalence in this population,[13,21] so these associations may not generalize to other groups.

Specifically, within college samples, certain characteristics have been reported to be linked to a higher risk of stimulant misuse (**Box 1**). Studies have found that misusers are more likely to have fraternity or sorority membership.[22] Additionally, several factors that predict low academic performance have been found to correlate with stimulant

Box 1
High-risk college groups for prescription stimulant misuse
White men
Attending colleges in the Northeast
Attending competitive colleges
Fraternity and sorority affiliation
Poor academic performance (low GPA, skipping class, etc.)
Substance use/SUD
Prominent ADHD symptoms and/or untreated ADHD
Poorer executive functioning and neuropsychological functioning

misuse, such as low grade point average (GPA), skipping class, and less time spent studying.[23,24]

Comorbidity with Stimulant Misuse

Stimulant misuse in TAY has been found to be associated with psychopathology. Among psychiatric disorders reported in stimulant misusers, depression,[25] conduct disorder,[26] ADHD, and SUD are the most well documented in the literature.[21,24,26]

ADHD symptoms, such as higher levels of inattention and impulsivity, are more commonly reported among stimulant misusers compared with individuals who do not misuse stimulants.[27,28] Stimulant misusers have also been shown to exhibit greater deficits on subjective measures of executive functioning as well as objective tests of neuropsychological functioning.[29] Compared with controls, misusers demonstrate lower academic performance,[23,24] not unlike those found in ADHD. Punctuating the authors' previous work,[26] Benson and colleagues[30] found that students with increased ADHD symptomology were almost 3 times more likely to misuse stimulants, even when controlling for comorbidity. Although this evidence suggests that untreated ADHD could be directly associated with stimulant misuse, further analysis has also suggested that co-occurring conduct disorder and/or SUD may play an important role in the link between ADHD and stimulant misuse.[17,31]

One of the most replicated findings in the literature is the strong association between stimulant misuse and substance use and SUD. Stimulants often are misused in the context of alcohol, marijuana, or other drugs use.[24] For instance, in a sample of 12,431 high school seniors surveyed, McCabe and colleagues[32] found that among past-year stimulant misusers (n = 835), 64% co-ingested stimulants with other substances, primarily alcohol and marijuana. Not surprisingly, high school seniors who misuse stimulants have been reported to be at higher risk for increased substance use.[33] Similar results have been found in undergraduate populations, with 1 study showing 46% of stimulant misusers reporting co-use with alcohol[34] and others reporting that misusers were more likely to engage in other substance use and polydrug use.[35] Furthermore, those who engaged in co-ingestion of stimulants and alcohol were more likely to report lower GPAs, use of other substances, and worse consequences compared with peers who ingested either substance in isolation.[34] The authors also reported that more than one-third of college-aged stimulant misusers actually met *Diagnostic and Statistical Manual of Mental Disorders, fourth edition,* criteria for either subthreshold or full-threshold stimulant use disorder, and one-half met criteria for an SUD.[26] Stimulant misuse in college students may also lead to long-term adverse effects. In a 17-year follow-up study (mean age 35 years at follow-up) using a national survey of 8362 high schoolers, McCabe and colleagues[36] found a higher likelihood of substance use and substance-related problems in those who misused stimulants in high school compared with students with no use or appropriate use of stimulants. Thus, it is important to evaluate individuals with misuse for other comorbidities.

Motivations

There is increasing evidence that stimulants frequently are misused for academic reasons or as a study aid.[37–39] A majority of motivations for stimulant misuse have consistently been found to include achieving better grades, increasing productivity, and improving alertness or concentration.[26,27] In some cases, self-treating underlying ADHD symptoms also has been reported as a motivation for misuse.[26,35] Although less frequent, other motivations, such as getting high, partying, or enhancing other drugs, also have been reported in TAY.[26,35,37,38]

COGNITIVE ENHANCEMENT

Even though self-reported motivations for stimulant misuse frequently include performance enhancement and as an academic aid, data regarding measurable positive cognitive effects in healthy individuals using stimulants remain inconclusive (**Table 1**). For instance, some studies in healthy adult volunteers given stimulants have reported increased measured spatial working memory,[40] planning,[41] error detection,[42] declarative memory consolidation,[43] and 5-choice continuous performance test.[44] Additionally, others have shown that those healthy individuals who benefit most from stimulants also demonstrated lower baseline cognitive performance.[45]

Weighed against the aforementioned positive findings, recent work has reported a nil effect of stimulants on cognitive performance. Recent controlled studies have reported subjective differences in cognition rather than objective cognitive enhancement, suggesting perceived effects may play a large role in stimulant misuse as opposed to truly enhanced cognitive performance. For example, in a small controlled trial, 13 college students without ADHD were given mixed-salts amphetamine, 30 mg, and then underwent assessments of neurocognition, mood, activation, and perceived cognitive enhancement.[46] Weyandt and colleagues[46] found minimal associations with neurocognitive enhancements (decreased working memory and improved attention); however, significant increases in subjective drug experience, activated positive emotion, and autonomic activity (heart rate and diastolic and systolic blood pressure) were observed. Although participants did not perceive enhanced cognitive abilities after stimulant administration, they did report perceived reduced previous performance relative to placebo administration. Similarly, college students who endorsed high-risk behavior associated with misuse showed increased perceived mood but not improved enhanced performance when expecting to receive methylphenidate (MPH) and instead receiving placebo.[47] In a controlled crossover study, comparing mixed-amphetamine salt, 10 mg, versus placebo, participants on active medication did not demonstrate enhanced cognitive performance.[48] Instead, participants who believed they had taken placebo performed worse on cognitive tasks on both placebo and active medication, whereas, when participants received active medication and believed they had taken active medication, their cognitive performance improved.[48] These findings highlight the potential influence of expectancy or of placebo response in cognitive enhancement experienced with stimulant misuse. Alternatively, the enhancement could be motivational in nature rather than cognitive, as demonstrated

Table 1

Representative studies of recent controlled studies of the cognitive enhancement effects of prescription stimulants

Study	Study Design	N	Age Range (y)	Stimulant	Dose	Cognitive Enhancement	Comments
Weyandt et al,[46] 2018	Double-blind, PBO-controlled, crossover	13	18–24	AMP	30 mg	Minimally improved attention performance (d = −0.17 – −0.73) and impaired working memory performance (d = 0.08–0.23)	Substantial effects on autonomic activity (d = 0.86–1.25; P<.001), subjective drug experience (d = 1.04–1.26; P<.01), and activated positive emotion (d = 0.71; P<.05)
MacQueen et al,[44] 2018	Double-blind, PBO-controlled, parallel	71	18–35	d-AMP	10 mg or 20 mg	Increased 5-choice continuous performance test for both doses in signal detection (d = 0.821, 0.758; P<.05) and response accuracy (d = 1.115 and 1.076; P<.001)	
Cropsey et al,[48] 2017	PBO-controlled, crossover	39	19–30	AMP	10 mg	None	Expecting medication was associated with cognitive enhancement and expecting placebo was associated with worse cognitive performance.
Agay et al,[45] 2014	PBO-controlled, crossover	39	20–40	MPH	0.3 mg/kg	Improved sustained attention (P<.05) and working memory (P<.01); no effects in decision making	Healthy individuals with lower baseline performance showed most improvement.
Linssen et al,[43] 2012	Double-blind, PBO-controlled, crossover	19	18–40	MPH	10 mg, 20 mg, or 40 mg	Dose-dependent improvement in memory consolidation (P<.05), set shifting (P<.05), and stopped signal performance (P<.01); no effects on spatial working memory or planning	
Looby & Earleywine,[47] 2011	Controlled, parallel (no active stimulant)	96	18–25	None	N/A	None	Expecting medication (blinded PBO) was associated with improved subjective mood (P<.01) vs no intervention.

All studies presented were randomized.

Abbreviations: AMP, mixed-salts amphetamine; d-AMP, dextroamphetamine; MPH, methylphenidate; PBO, placebo.

in a pilot study that found that the strongest subjective effects misusers reported in a self-report survey were improvements in alertness and energy and not in other cognitive abilities.[49] These data support meta-analytic findings of inconsistent neurocognitive enhancement effects of prescription stimulants in the literature, concluding that stimulants caused no effects on planning accuracy and optimal decision making and resulted only in potential improvements in processing speed in healthy adults.[50] Based on the literature, it seems that stimulant use in healthy individuals may produce mild cognitive enhancement, with the major confounds of expectations of cognitive enhancement with stimulants. Given the limited sample sizes, variability in outcome measures, and issues with differentiation of expectancy from objective outcomes, further research in this area is necessary.

CONSEQUENCES OF STIMULANT MISUSE

Nonmedical use of stimulants can lead to adverse short-term and longer-term outcomes. Besides common side effects of stimulants that also could occur in stimulant misuse, such as decreased appetite, insomnia, irritability, headaches, and stomachaches,[51] stimulants can cause an increase in heart rate and blood pressure, which may lead to adverse cardiovascular effects, especially in those with underlying conditions, such as high blood pressure, that are not screened as part of therapeutic administration. The lack of medical oversight during nonmedical use can lead to more severe outcomes due to risky behaviors, such as ingestion of high doses or with other substances, intranasal administration, or misuse by individuals with contraindications to stimulants.

The consequences of stimulant misuse are further demonstrated by the recent, significant increase in emergency department visits related to nonmedical stimulant misuse—tripling between 2005 and 2010[52]—and often linked to the use of stimulants and other substances simultaneously.[53] Mattson[54] found that in emergency department visits related to nonmedical stimulant use, other pharmaceutical drugs, illicit drugs, and alcohol were related in 45%, 21%, and 19% of visits respectively, highlighting the potential serious adverse effects of co-use of stimulant use and other substances.

Furthermore, when administered intranasally, prescription stimulants have been shown to have higher abuse liability and higher risk of cardiovascular effects[55] relative to oral administration. Although several studies have found that most students report oral use of stimulants,[38] a substantial minority of individuals use stimulants intranasally.[6] For instance, the authors recently reported that 38% of college students misused stimulants intranasally.[56] Intranasal administration has been found to be associated with co-ingestion of other substances and recreational motives compared with oral administration.[32] Additionally, the effects of intranasal stimulant misuse occur rapidly within minutes of administration compared with the slower onset (up to 1 hour) in oral administration, resulting in an increased abuse liability and similarities with the consequences of cocaine use (for review, see Sussman and colleagues[57]).

DISCUSSION: STRATEGIES TO MITIGATE AND PREVENT STIMULANT MISUSE AND DIVERSION

Because primary motivations for stimulant misuse are academic in nature and subjective cognitive enhancement seems to play a substantial role in stimulant misuse, it is important to portray accurate information about the potential consequences of misuse. Students misusing stimulants believe that taking stimulants will improve their grades,[27,39] and most misusers report perceiving misuse as widespread and not associated with negative consequences to physical or mental health.[58] Thus, individual prescribers and programs on college campuses that educate about these misperceptions and highlight the potential consequences of high-risk behavior and administration are necessary. Prevention efforts aimed at students who could be struggling academically should include accessible academic resources and support.

Additionally, when treating college-aged patients, it is helpful to consider behaviors and subgroups at risk for misuse and markers of more severe stimulant misuse. For example, evaluating methods of misuse may provide insight into the likelihood of other risky behavior and other substance use. Regarding treatment, practitioners may find that certain treatment plans could be enhanced, depending on any additional comorbidities identified. Stimulant misusers with ADHD symptoms may benefit from an evaluation and treatment of ADHD, increased academic support, and education on the risks of stimulant misuse. Misusers with SUD should be considered for full evaluation and treatment, including psychotherapy and/or pharmacotherapy, in order to evaluate and stabilize their SUD and accompanying comorbidities.

In cases of TAY patients presenting for ADHD, several guidelines have been posited that may reduce the likelihood of stimulant misuse and diversion. The provider must first consider if the patient is malingering to obtain medication. If there is any suspicion regarding a recent diagnosis, the provider can evaluate the patient in a more comprehensive, multistep process that includes requesting and assessing past records and lengthening the prescribing process, discouraging individuals seeking stimulants for nonmedical reasons.

If an ADHD diagnosis is confirmed and pharmacotherapy is initiated, conversations between the prescriber and patient should include clear instructions for proper administration and storage of medication and education regarding misuse and diversion. Providers should consider carefully which medication type and preparation are most appropriate when working with TAY. Prescribers are advised to screen adolescents and young adults with ADHD for substance use and SUD, because TAY who misuse alcohol, marijuana, or other substances are more likely to divert or misuse their own stimulant medication than non–substance-using peers.[59] For TAY patients with ADHD and comorbid SUD, nonstimulants, such as atomoxetine, bupropion, and tricyclic antidepressants, may be considered due to their lower abuse liability.[60] When considering stimulants, differences exist in abuse liability, with extended-release stimulants having lower abuse liability compared with equipotent doses of immediate-release stimulants,[61] resulting in less misuse and diversion of the extended-release compared with immediate-release preparations.[26] In addition to lower abuse liability, extended-release stimulants provide the benefit of consistent treatment to TAY throughout the day.[59]

When working with TAY with ADHD, providers should pay careful attention to possible misuse or diversion by monitoring pill counts, prescribing only the amount of medication necessary, and recognizing premature refill requests. Excess supplies of stimulant medication represent one of the largest sources of diverted, and subsequently misused, stimulants.[13] Querying about substance use and SUD should be considered at follow-up visits, with toxicology testing in those suspected of manifesting a SUD. Clinicians also are encouraged to provide patients and parents with instructions on safe storage (eg, not in medicine cabinets) and education regarding the medical, psychological, ethical, and legal consequences of misuse and diversion.

SUMMARY

Stimulants used to treat ADHD currently are the most common prescription medications used nonmedically in young people. Stimulant misuse is associated with other psychiatric comorbidities, such as ADHD and SUD, as well as academic underachievement, neuropsychological dysfunction, and continued impairment longer term. Due to the pervasive nature of stimulant misuse among adolescents and young adults, particularly on college campuses, prescribers should evaluate individuals for risk factors of misuse as well as educate and monitor for misuse or diversion. Young people with stimulant misuse should be evaluated for routes of misuse, behavioral disorders and SUD, and neuropsychological and academic dysfunction. Although the literature has not reached a consensus regarding the cognitive effects of ADHD stimulant use in healthy individuals, it seems that subjective effects might play a substantial role in perceived cognitive enhancement. Despite the wealth of information now available on stimulant misuse, additional research is necessary on prevention efforts to mitigate stimulant misuse, treatment strategies for those with stimulant misuse, and safer stimulant preparations.

DISCLOSURE

Dr T.E. Wilens is codirector of the Center for Addiction Medicine at Massachusetts General Hospital. He receives grant support from the following sources: NIH (NIDA). Dr T.E. Wilens has published a book, *Straight Talk about Psychiatric Medications for Kids* (Guilford Press), and coedited books, *Attention-Deficit Hyperactivity Disorder in Adults and Children* (Cambridge University Press), *Massachusetts General Hospital Comprehensive Clinical Psychiatry* (Elsevier), and *Massachusetts General Hospital Psychopharmacology and Neurotherapeutics* (Elsevier). Dr T.E. Wilens is co-owner of a copyrighted diagnostic questionnaire (Before School Functioning Questionnaire) and has a licensing agreement with Ironshore (BSFQ Questionnaire). He is or has been a consultant for Alcobra, KemPharm, Otsuka, and Ironshore and serves as a clinical consultant to the National Football League (ERM Associates), Minor/Major League Baseball, Gavin Foundation, and Bay Cove Human Services. T.A. Kaminski has no conflicts of interest to disclose.

REFERENCES

1. Merikangas KR, He JP, Burstein M, et al. Service utilization for lifetime mental disorders in U.S. adolescents: results of the National Comorbidity Survey-Adolescent Supplement (NCS-A). J Am Acad Child Adolesc Psychiatry 2011; 50(1):32–45.

2. Ascherman LI, Shaftel J. Facilitating transition from high school and special education to adult life: focus on youth with learning disorders, attention-deficit/hyperactivity disorder, and speech/language impairments. Child Adolesc Psychiatr Clin N Am 2017;26(2):311–27.

3. Stevens JR, Wilens TE, Stern TA. Using stimulants for attention-deficit/hyperactivity disorder: clinical approaches and challenges. Prim Care Companion 2013;15(2):1–12.

4. Wilens TE, Isenberg BM, Kaminski TA, et al. Attention-deficit/hyperactivity disorder and transitional aged youth. Curr Psychiatry Rep 2018;20(11):100.

5. McCabe SE, Teter CJ, Boyd CJ. Medical use, illicit use and diversion of prescription stimulant medication. J Psychoactive Drugs 2006;38(1):43–56.

6. Garnier-Dykstra LM, Caldeira KM, Vincent KB, et al. Nonmedical use of prescription stimulants during college: four-year trends in exposure opportunity, use, motives, and sources. J Am Coll Health 2012;60(3):226–34.

7. Miesch M, Deister A. Attention-deficit/hyperactivity disorder (ADHD) in adult psychiatry: data on 12-month prevalence, risk factors and comorbidity. Fortschr Neurol Psychiatr 2018;87(1):32–8 [in German].

8. McCabe SE, Dickinson K, West BT, et al. Age of onset, duration, and type of medication therapy for attention-deficit/hyperactivity disorder and substance use during adolescence: a multi-cohort national study. J Am Acad Child Adolesc Psychiatry 2016;55(6):479–86.

9. Quinn PD, Chang Z, Hur K, et al. ADHD medication and substance-related problems. Am J Psychiatry 2017;174(9):877–85.

10. Wilens TE, McKowen J, Kane M. Transitional-aged youth and substance use: teenaged addicts come of age. Contemp Pediatr 2013;30(11):24–30.

11. Quality CfBHSa. 2017 National survey on drug use and health: detailed tables. Rockville (MD): Substance Abuse and Mental Health Services Administration; 2018.

12. Schepis TS, Wilens TE, McCabe SE. Prescription drug misuse: sources of controlled medications in adolescents. J Am Acad Child Adolesc Psychiatry 2019;58(7):670–80.e4.

13. McCabe SE, Teter CJ, Boyd CJ, et al. Sources of prescription medication misuse among young adults in the United States: the role of educational status. J Clin Psychiatry 2018;79(2) [pii:17m11958].

14. Epstein-Ngo QM, McCabe SE, Veliz PT, et al. Diversion of ADHD stimulants and victimization among adolescents. J Pediatr Psychol 2016;41(7):786–98.

15. Gallucci AR, Martin RJ, Usdan SL. The diversion of stimulant medications among a convenience sample of college students with current prescriptions. Psychol Addict Behav 2015;29(1):154–61.

16. McCabe SE, West BT, Cranford JA, et al. Medical misuse of controlled medications among adolescents. Arch Pediatr Adolesc Med 2011;165(8):729–35.

17. Wilens T, Gignac M, Swezey A, et al. Characteristics of adolescents and young adults with ADHD who divert or misuse their prescribed medications. J Am Acad Child Adolesc Psychiatry 2006;45(4):408–14.

18. Benson K, Flory K, Humphreys KL, et al. Misuse of stimulant medication among college students: a comprehensive review and meta-analysis. Clin Child Fam Psychol Rev 2015;18(1):50–76.

19. Cruz S, Sumstine S, Mendez J, et al. Health-compromising practices of undergraduate college students: Examining racial/ethnic and gender differences in characteristics of prescription stimulant misuse. Addict Behav 2017;68:59–65.

20. Wu LT, Schlenger WE. Psychostimulant dependence in a community sample. Subst Use Misuse 2003;38(2):221–48.

21. McCabe SE, Knight JR, Teter CJ, et al. Non-medical use of prescription stimulants among US college students: prevalence and correlates from a national survey. Addiction 2005;100(1):96–106.

22. Dussault CL, Weyandt LL. An examination of prescription stimulant misuse and psychological variables among sorority and fraternity college populations. J Atten Disord 2013;17(2):87–97.

23. Rabiner DL, Anastopoulos AD, Costello EJ, et al. Motives and perceived consequences of nonmedical ADHD medication use by college students: are students treating themselves for attention problems? J Atten Disord 2009;13(3):259–70.

24. Arria AM, Wilcox HC, Caldeira KM, et al. Dispelling the myth of "smart drugs": cannabis and alcohol use problems predict nonmedical use of prescription stimulants for studying. Addict Behav 2013;38(3):1643–50.

25. Poulin C. From attention-deficit/hyperactivity disorder to medical stimulant use to the diversion of prescribed stimulants to non-medical stimulant use: connecting the dots. Addiction 2007;102(5):740–51.

26. Wilens T, Zulauf C, Martelon M, et al. Nonmedical stimulant use in college students: association with attention-deficit/hyperactivity disorder and other disorders. J Clin Psychiatry 2016;77(7):940–7.

27. Peterkin AL, Crone CC, Sheridan MJ, et al. Cognitive performance enhancement: misuse or self-treatment? J Atten Disord 2011;15(4):263–8.

28. Looby A, Sant'Ana S. Nonmedical prescription stimulant users experience subjective but not objective impairments in attention and impulsivity. Am J Addict 2018;27(3):238–44.

29. Wilens TE, Carrellas NW, Martelon M, et al. Neuropsychological functioning in college students who misuse prescription stimulants. Am J Addict 2017;26(4): 379–87.

30. Benson K, Woodlief DT, Flory K, et al. Is ADHD, independent of ODD, associated with whether and why college students misuse stimulant medication? Exp Clin Psychopharmacol 2018;26(5):476–87.

31. Brook JS, Balka EB, Zhang C, et al. ADHD, conduct disorder, substance use disorder, and nonprescription stimulant use. J Atten Disord 2017;21(9):776–82.

32. McCabe SE, West BT, Schepis TS, et al. Simultaneous co-ingestion of prescription stimulants, alcohol and other drugs: a multi-cohort national study of US adolescents. Hum Psychopharmacol 2015;30(1):42–51.

33. Teter CJ, DiRaimo CG, West BT, et al. Nonmedical use of prescription stimulants among US high school students to help study: results from a national survey. J Pharm Pract 2018. 897190018783887.

34. Egan KL, Reboussin BA, Blocker JN, et al. Simultaneous use of non-medical ADHD prescription stimulants and alcohol among undergraduate students. Drug Alcohol Depend 2013;131(1–2):71–7.

35. Rabiner DL, Anastopoulos AD, Costello EJ, et al. The misuse and diversion of prescribed ADHD medications by college students. J Atten Disord 2009;13(2): 144–53.

36. McCabe SE, Veliz P, Wilens TE, et al. Adolescents' prescription stimulant use and adult functional outcomes: a national prospective study. J Am Acad Child Adolesc Psychiatry 2017;56(3):226–33.e4.

37. Teter CJ, McCabe SE, LaGrange K, et al. Illicit use of specific prescription stimulants among college students: prevalence, motives, and routes of administration. Pharmacotherapy 2006;26(10):1501–10.

38. Bavarian N, McMullen J, Flay BR, et al. A mixed-methods approach examining illicit prescription stimulant use: findings from a Northern California University. J Prim Prev 2017;38(4):363–83.

39. Arria AM, Geisner IM, Cimini MD, et al. Perceived academic benefit is associated with nonmedical prescription stimulant use among college students. Addict Behav 2018;76:27–33.

40. Mehta MA, Owen AM, Sahakian BJ, et al. Methylphenidate enhances working memory by modulating discrete frontal and parietal lobe regions in the human brain. J Neurosci 2000;20(6):RC65.

41. Elliott R, Sahakian BJ, Matthews K, et al. Effects of methylphenidate on spatial working memory and planning in healthy young adults. Psychopharmacology (Berl) 1997;131(2):196–206.

42. Hester R, Nandam LS, O'Connell RG, et al. Neurochemical enhancement of conscious error awareness. J Neurosci 2012;32(8):2619–27.

43. Linssen AM, Vuurman EF, Sambeth A, et al. Methylphenidate produces selective enhancement of declarative memory consolidation in healthy volunteers. Psychopharmacology (Berl) 2012;221(4):611–9.

44. MacQueen DA, Minassian A, Kenton JA, et al. Amphetamine improves mouse and human attention in the 5-choice continuous performance test. Neuropharmacology 2018;138:87–96.

45. Agay N, Yechiam E, Carmel Z, et al. Methylphenidate enhances cognitive performance in adults with poor baseline capacities regardless of attention-deficit/hyperactivity disorder diagnosis. J Clin Psychopharmacol 2014;34(2):261–5.

46. Weyandt LL, White TL, Gudmundsdottir BG, et al. Neurocognitive, autonomic, and mood effects of adderall: a pilot study of healthy college students. Pharmacy (Basel) 2018;6(3) [pii:E58].

47. Looby A, Earleywine M. Expectation to receive methylphenidate enhances subjective arousal but not cognitive performance. Exp Clin Psychopharmacol 2011;19(6):433–44.

48. Cropsey KL, Schiavon S, Hendricks PS, et al. Mixed-amphetamine salts expectancies among college students: Is stimulant induced cognitive enhancement a placebo effect? Drug Alcohol Depend 2017;178:302–9.

49. Ilieva IP, Farah MJ. Enhancement stimulants: perceived motivational and cognitive advantages. Front Neurosci 2013;7:198.

50. Marraccini ME, Weyandt LL, Rossi JS, et al. Neurocognitive enhancement or impairment? A systematic meta-analysis of prescription stimulant effects on processing speed, decision-making, planning, and cognitive perseveration. Exp Clin Psychopharmacol 2016;24(4):269–84.

51. Advokat CD, Guidry D, Martino L. Licit and illicit use of medications for Attention-Deficit Hyperactivity Disorder in undergraduate college students. J Am Coll Health 2008;56(6):601–6.

52. Substance Abuse and Mental Health Services Administration CfBHSaQ. The DAWN Report: emergency department visits involving attention deficit/hyperactivity disorder stimulant medications. Rockville, MD, January 24, 2013. 2013.

53. Chen LY, Crum RM, Strain EC, et al. Prescriptions, nonmedical use, and emergency department visits involving prescription stimulants. J Clin Psychiatry 2016;77(3):e297–304.

54. Mattson ME. Emergency department visits involving attention deficit/hyperactivity disorder stimulant medications. Rockville (MD): The CBHSQ report; 2013. p. 1–8.

55. Stoops WW, Glaser PE, Rush CR. Reinforcing, subject-rated, and hysiological effects of intranasal methylphenidate in humans: a dose-response analysis. Drug Alcohol Depend 2003;71(2):179–86.

56. Wilens TE, Martelon M, Yule A, et al. Disentangling the context of stimulant misuse in college students. 65th Annual Meetings of the Am Acad Child Adolesc Psychiatry. Seattle, Washington, October 22-27, 2018.

57. Sussman S, Pentz MA, Spruijt-Metz D, et al. Misuse of "study drugs:" prevalence, consequences, and implications for policy. Subst Abuse Treat Prev Policy 2006;1:15.

58. Kilmer JR, Geisner IM, Gasser ML, et al. Normative perceptions of non-medical stimulant use: associations with actual use and hazardous drinking. Addict Behav 2015;42:51–6.

59. Wilens T, Carrellas N, Biederman J. ADHD and substance misuse. In: Banaschewski T, editor. Oxford textbook of attention deficit hyperactivity disorder. New York: Oxford University Press; 2016. p. 215–26.

60. Colaneri N, Keim S, Adesman A. Physician practices to prevent ADHD stimulant diversion and misuse. J Subst Abuse Treat 2017;74:26–34.

61. Spencer TJ, Biederman J, Ciccone PE, et al. PET study examining pharmacokinetics, detection and likeability, and dopamine transporter receptor occupancy of short- and long-acting oral methylphenidate. Am J Psychiatry 2006;163(3): 387–95.

Focus on Adolescent Use of Club Drugs and "Other" Substances

Janet F. Williams, MD[a],*, Leslie H. Lundahl, PhD[b]

KEYWORDS

- Adolescents • Club drugs • Designer drugs • Hallucinogens • Inhalants
- OTC substances • SBIRT

KEY POINTS

- Despite decreases in use, club drugs and "other" drugs will remain among the evolving and diverse selection of abusable substances used by adolescents.
- Adolescents most often use the least expensive, most accessible substances they perceive to have the lowest risk.
- Potential users and health care providers should remain highly suspicious about the content or purity of any of this article's substances being one specific drug or drug class.
- Health care providers should be prepared for club and other drug users to come to medical attention most often through acute or emergency presentations.
- Health care practitioners caring for adolescents must stay well-informed about practice area drug use trends, and specific substance use-related health effects and presentations for care.

The category of "other" abuseable substances sought by adolescents and young adults continues to evolve and includes diverse substances and drug classes, particularly club drugs, dissociative anesthetics, hallucinogens, inhalants, and over-the-counter substances. This article offers a brief update of the authors' 2014 detailed review of the epidemiology, detection, presentation, and acute and long-term management considerations when adolescents use dextromethorphan (DXM), flunitrazepam (Rohypnol), gamma-hydroxybutyrate (GHB), inhalants, ketamine, lysergic acid diethylamide (LSD), methylenedioxymethamphetamine (MDMA), phencyclidine, *Salvia divinorum* (salvia), synthetic cannabinoids, and/or synthetic cathinones (bath salts).[1]

Disclosure Statement: J.F. Williams - Nothing to disclose regarding relationship with a commercial company with direct financial interest as stated. L.H. Lundahl – Nothing to disclose.
[a] Department of Pediatrics, Long School of Medicine, University of Texas Health San Antonio, 7703 Floyd Curl Drive, MD 7802, San Antonio, TX 78229-3900, USA; [b] Substance Abuse Research Division, Department of Psychiatry and Behavioral Neurosciences, Wayne State University School of Medicine, 3901 Chrysler Service Drive, Suite 2A, Detroit, MI 48201, USA
* Corresponding author.
E-mail address: jawilliams@uthscsa.edu

INTRODUCTION

The cluster of "other" substances used by adolescents and young adults includes substances classified as club drugs, dissociative anesthetics, hallucinogens, and/or inhalants, but this categorization does not fully reveal the diversity of the drugs within any 1 class in terms of pharmacology, effects and routes of use. The "club drug" label arose about 3 decades ago when a recognizable drug use pattern emerged among regular patrons of nightclubs and *raves* or all-night dance parties. Stimulant club drugs promote staying awake all night and hallucinatory effects with intense feelings of elation, well-being, and sensory awareness, while sedative club drugs ease "coming down" from the high. Six drugs—flunitrazepam, GHB, ketamine, LSD, MDMA (Ecstasy or Molly), and methamphetamine—were identified by the National Institute on Drug Abuse as club drugs, and the first 3 of these are also called predatory or "date rape" drugs.[2]

Any synthetic derivative of a federally controlled substance that has been produced clandestinely and illegally for illicit use is popularly called a "designer drug." The term "designer" indicates the drug was specifically created through slight alteration of the original drug's molecular structure. The variety of ways to categorize drugs means that several of the club drugs and "other" substances of abuse discussed here also belong to more than one category. For example, ketamine is both a dissociative and a club drug; Ecstasy is a designer drug, club drug, and hallucinogen as well as a stimulant. Much inhalant use is abuse of an over-the-counter (OTC) substance just like DXM abuse. Salvia is an abusable natural plant-based substance from the mint family[2,3] that also has dissociative and hallucinogen effects.

Because so many factors impact the extent of "other" substance abuse by adolescents and young adults, the type of drugs available and frequency of use will continue to evolve. Some of these impacting factors are the actual and the perceived substance availability, the perceived benefits or risk of use, generational memory or "forgetting" of adverse consequences, substance legalization or regulatory reclassification, new drug forms or new drug delivery devices, and the continued production of new abusable chemicals by designer drug laboratories.

EPIDEMIOLOGY

The annual Monitoring the Future (MTF) survey and other research continue to show that current adolescent and young adult use prevalence rates for any illicit substances are much lower than peak use rates in earlier decades.[4–8] **Table 1** shows the MTF 2018 rates of past-year use by US adolescents.[4]

Although sex differences in substance use have narrowed as use prevalence has decreased, males continue to have somewhat higher rates of illicit drug use, and notably higher rates of frequent use, particularly by 12th grade. Conversely, in 8th grade, inhalant and amphetamine use is higher in females.[4–6]

Similar to any substance use, "other" substance use crosses every sociodemographic boundary and occurs in all regions of the United States, remote and high population areas, and among all ethnic groups. Illicit substance use prevalence has been shifting among the 3 largest racial/ethnic groups surveyed through MTF—white, African American, Hispanic. White students compared with African American students have for years had substantially higher illicit drug use rates, but marijuana use has increased among African American students of all ages, so that group's overall illicit drug use rate now resembles that of the others. African American students continue to have lower use of hallucinogens, synthetic marijuana, and all forms of prescription drugs without a prescription, but bath salt use has exceeded use by whites or

Table 1
MTF: Prevalence of annual substance use

	12th Graders		10th Graders	8th Graders
	Peak Annual	2018 Annual	2018 Annual	2018 Annual
DXM	6.9	3.4	3.3	2.8
GHB	2	0.3	Not asked	Not asked
Inhalants	8	1.6	2.4	4.6
Ketamine	2.6	0.7	Not asked	Not asked
LSD	8.8	3.2	2.0	0.9
MDMA (Ecstasy, Molly)	9.2	2.2	1.4	1.1
Rohypnol	1.6	0.7	0.3	0.3
Salvia	5.9	0.9	0.7	0.6
Synthetic cannabinoids	11.4	3.5	2.9	1.6
Synthetic cathinones (bath salts)	1.3	0.6	0.5	0.9

Annual = Percent who reported "use in past year."
Data from Johnston LD, Miech RA, O'Malley PM, et al. Monitoring the Future national survey results on drug use, 1975-2018: overview, key findings on adolescent drug use. Ann Arbor: Institute for Social Research, University of Michigan. Available at: http://www.monitoringthefuture.org/. Accessed March 1, 2019.

Hispanics. In 8th grade, Hispanics generally report the highest use rates of nearly all drug classes, and in 12th grade, continue to have the highest use rates for synthetic marijuana, crystal methamphetamine and forms of cocaine. Any inexpensive and highly accessible substance of abuse, such as inhalants or alcohol, has a greater use prevalence among adolescents in general, but particularly among geographically isolated populations experiencing impoverished living conditions, such as American Indian youth living on a reservation or otherwise isolated.

RECENT DRUG USE TRENDS

By 2018, the annual 12th-grade use prevalence of Rohypnol, GHB, ketamine, and PCP had all decreased by at least one-half compared with peak use prevalences about 20 years earlier. Since inclusion in the 2000 MTF survey, GHB and ketamine annual use rates for all grades had trended low enough by 2012 to warrant discontinuing those questions for 8th and 10th graders. MDMA, mostly known for years as Ecstasy, has shown variable use trends and been popular more for its mildly hallucinogenic properties than its stimulant effects. Use prevalence in all 3 grades has decreased since 2016. By 2013, Molly had sufficient popularity for the 2014 MTF questions to include that term to help explain use trends. Molly is slang for "molecular," a term that was coined to indicate pure MDMA, because Ecstasy was becoming known to contain additives, such as caffeine and methamphetamine, and losing popularity. Molly itself has since been reported to be adulterated with harmful substances, particularly synthetic cathinones. In 2018, salvia continued to gradually decrease to such low use that MTF may discontinue those questions.[4] The use prevalence of DXM, a cough suppressant found in many OTC cough and cold preparations, has halved since MTF survey inclusion in 2006.[4]

Substances classified as inhalants comprise a large and pharmacologically diverse group of noncombusted and nonheated volatile chemicals that are inhaled with the intent to achieve an altered mental state. Inhalants do not attract as much attention from media or health professionals compared with "other" drugs, despite being a more prevalent problem, so inhalant use remains largely under-recognized. Both the MTF and the National Survey on Drug Use and Health studies have demonstrated how inhalant use differs from "other" drug use, which most notably is that use consistently decreases with advancing age.[4–6,8] Volatile products are widely available, inexpensive, easily concealed, and legal for intended purposes, such as household aerosol products. These factors all contribute to greater use by younger age groups. Much of the decline in use with age has already occurred by 10th grade, and there is very little inhalant use by age 20 years.[4–6,8] Inhalant use is slightly higher among girls in grades 8 and 10, but boys show higher rates by grade 12 and thereafter.[4,7]

Both LSD and inhalants are excellent examples of drugs that undergo "generational forgetting," such that over time, younger generations less knowledgeable about a drug's effects periodically "rediscover" both the desired effects and the associated risk. Annual questions about perceived risk and disapproval of use inform trends inversely related to use prevalence trends. Greater percentages of young adolescents have in recent years responded "can't say, drug unfamiliar" to questions about risk and disapproval of LSD use, potentially portending a resurgence.[4]

DETECTION

All patient populations include substance users, so all health care providers should stay well-informed about local and wider drug use trends, and the most common manner in which popular drugs are used (**Table 2**).[2,9–11] Current substance use and addiction knowledge and skills are needed to practice routine and effective patient care screening, recognition, and management of substance use. Validated, age-appropriate Screening, Brief Intervention and referral to Treatment (SBIRT) tools promote rapid and confidential clinical approaches to ascertain drug use and demonstrate adoption of responsive best practices.[12,13] The following important considerations are relevant to substance use detection whether based on the patient's presenting signs and symptoms or the laboratory drug testing usually conducted on urine or blood samples.

- Suspicion that an adolescent may be using *any* substance, particularly illicit or OTC substances, should raise concern for possible multiple drug use, because unintentional use of multiple substances is as common as intentional use.
- The use of multiple substances may present with nonspecific symptoms, or with mixed or potentiated symptomatology (eg, when a depressant drug or inhalant is used with alcohol).
- Drug popularity varies by region, availability, and access.
- Drug testing methods and routine laboratory screening panels used by hospitals and reference laboratories have known technological limits and may vary by locale.[3,14,15]
- Urine drug testing is the gold standard but does not detect DXM, GHB, inhalants, LSD, synthetic cannabinoids, synthetic cathinones, or salvia. Ketamine is not in the test panel.
- Rohypnol or MDMA are difficult to detect in urine because low dose use is common.
- Gas chromatography and mass spectrometry used in forensic testing can detect GHB, inhalants, LSD, Rohypnol and most "other" drugs, including metabolites of certain synthetic cannabinoids.[3,14,15]

Table 2
Common methods of substance use

	DXM	GHB	Inhalants	Ketamine	LSD	MDMA	Rohypnol	Salvia	Syn Cann	Syn Cath
Tablet/pill	X	X		X	X	X[a]	X			X
Liquid	X[a]	X		X	X	X	X			X
Dissolve		X[a]					X[a]			
Snort				X[a]		X	X			X[a]
Inject				X		X	X			X
Smoke/vape				X		X	X	X[a]	X[a]	
Inhale			X[a]							
Brew tea								X	X	
Chew dry or raw								X		
Blotter: treated paper in mouth					X[a]					

[a] Most common method of use.
Data from Refs.[2,9–11]

- Other laboratory testing can inform about acute or chronic substance use effects and detect concurrent abuse of multiple substances

SELECTED STREET, SLANG, AND CODE NAMES

Substances of abuse commonly acquire street names, slang or code names,[9–11] which vary among different US regions, states, cities and locales, but also within a single urban area. Street names commonly change to a few preferred terms through evolution over time, or to correspond with a real or implied substance preparation change. Common street names are presented in **Table 3**.

FEATURES COMMON TO VARIOUS CLUB DRUGS AND "OTHER" SUBSTANCES OF ABUSE

- The 3 classic date rape drugs have central nervous system depressant effects: GHB, ketamine, and Rohypnol.[1,2]
- *Designer drugs*: Amphetamine analogs like MDMA (Ecstasy and Molly), synthetic cannabinoids, and synthetic cathinones (bath salts)

Table 3 Selected street names	
Substance Name	**Selected Slang Terms and Code Words**
DXM	Dex, Red Devils, Red Hots, Robo, *Robotrip*, *Triple C*, Vitamin D
GHB	Blowout, Cherry Meth, Easy Lay, Fantasy, G, Gamma Oh, Georgia Home Boy, Goop, Grievous Bodily Harm, Jib, *Liquid E*, Liquid X, Monkey Juice, Salty Water, *Scoop*, *Soap*
Inhalants: volatile solvents, fuels and anesthetics	Air Blast, *Dust Off*, *Hippie Crack*, Moon Gas, Oz, Poor Man's Pot
Inhalants: nitrous oxide	*Laughing Gas*, *Whippets*
Inhalants: volatile alkyl nitrite	Amys, Bolt, Climax, Locker Room, *Poppers*, *Rush*, Thrust
Ketamine	Cat Valium, Donkey, Jet K, *Kit Kat*, *Special K*, Wonky
LSD	*Acid*, *Blotter*, Cube, Bomba, Cid, Dots, Elefante Blanco, Hits, *Microdot*, Orange Micros, Purple Haze, Sugar Cubes, Superman, Yellow Sunshine, Zen
MDMA	Adam, Beans, Bombs, Clarity, Disco Biscuits, *E*, *Ecstasy*, Essence, Eve, Green Apple, Hug, Love Drug, Lovers' Speed, Malcolm X, *Molly*, Peace, Pingaz, Thizz, Vowels, *X*, XTC
Rohypnol (flunitrazepam)	542, Circles, Date Rape Drug, *Forget Me Pill*, La Rocha, Lunch Money, *Mexican Valium*, Mind Eraser, Pingus, R2, Roach, Roachas, *Roofies*, Rope, Trip-and-Fall,
Salvia (*Salvia Divinorum*)	Diviner's Sage, Magic Mint, Maria Pastora, *Sally D*
Synthetic cannabinoids	Black Mamba, Bliss, Bombay Blue, Fire, Genie, Joker, *K2*, Kaos, OMG, Ninja, Pow, *Spice*, Yucatan Fire, Zohai
Synthetic cathinones	Bath Blow, *Bath Salts*, Bloom, Bliss, Bubbles, Cloud9, Ivory Wave, Lunar Wave, Plant Feeder, Salting, Scarface, Snow Leopard, Stardust, Vanilla Sky, White Lightning, Wicked X

Data from Refs.[9–11]

- *Dependence and withdrawal* symptoms: DXM, GHB, inhalants, ketamine, MDMA, synthetic cannabinoids, and synthetic cathinones
- *Dissociative effects:* DXM, ketamine, and salvia
- *Flashbacks*: DXM, ketamine, and LSD
- *Hallucinations, illusory or distorted perceptions*: DXM (visual/auditory hallucinations), GHB (visual/auditory hallucinations), inhalants, ketamine, LSD, MDMA (illusory distortions), Rohypnol, salvia, synthetic cathinones, and synthetic cannabinoids
- *Hyperthermia*: DXM and MDMA
- *Muscle rigidity, myoclonic spasms, grimacing bruxism, rhabdomyolysis*: GHB and MDMA
- *Psychosis with no prior history:* GHB (acute psychosis), chronic inhalant use, LSD, chronic MDMA use (paranoid schizophrenia), salvia (psychosis mimic), and synthetic cathinones (paranoia, panic)
- *Tolerance* with chronic use: DXM, GHB, inhalants, ketamine, LSD, and Rohypnol
- When providing care for a patient with suspected or known substance intoxication, the following points are important:
  ○ All intoxicated patients respond best in a calm, supportive, low-stimulation environment.
  ○ Always consider the need for decontamination of the patient's skin and clothing, and provider protection from contamination.
- Rapid consultation with clinical toxicology experts and/or a regional Poison Control Center can confirm any specifically indicated or contraindicated management approaches, particularly medication use.

DISTINCTIVE FEATURES BY DRUG

The diversity of club drugs and "other" abusable substances on the market should indicate to users and health care practitioners that there is a potential plethora of use-related effects to be anticipated other than the underlying desired effects for using the substance. Additionally, when multiple drugs are used together or similarly acting substances potentiate "other" drug effects, the results are manifest as discordant, similar, or mixed symptomatology. Most users reach medical health care attention through an acute or emergency setting owing to drug-related toxic effects still being experienced or secondary injury related to the substance having caused neurobehavioral changes that skewed the user's ability to interact safely with their surroundings. The medical history and physical examination are crucial to ascertaining and maneuvering the correct patient diagnostic and management pathways. The eyes are considered a direct extension of the central nervous system, and offer an accessible window to the brain. Any reported visual effects as well as eye findings documented through physical examination may offer pathognomonic or diagnostic findings before laboratory testing can be completed (**Table 4**).

DEXTROMETHORPHAN

DXM is the semisynthetic morphine derivative and active ingredient in more than 100 OTC cough and cold preparations.[1–3,11,16,17] When taken in doses much higher than recommended for cough, DXM acts as a dissociative drug with highly dose-dependent effects. Lower doses produce alertness, empathy, laughing, euphoria, and mild intoxication with tachycardia and temperature elevation; increased doses cause increased intensity of those effects plus hallucinations, mild dissociation, and a dreamlike state. Even higher doses cause loss of coordination, ataxia, a

Table 4
Classic eye findings on physical examination and reported vision changes

	Pupil Size	Gaze	Eye Position or Movement	Conjunctivae	Vision	Other Visual Disturbances
DXM	Mydriasis		Nystagmus		Blurred	Altered perceptions; dreamlike vision; perceived blindness
GBH	Mydriasis or Miosis; Pupillary light reflexes lost in deep coma		Nystagmus		Blurred with mydriasis; peripheral vision loss	
Inhalants				Injection, watering eyes	Diplopia	Visual hallucinations with prolonged use
Ketamine	Mydriasis	Fixed, sightless stare			Blurred or distorted vision	Visual distortions
LSD	Mydriasis				Blurred	Visual hallucinations Flashbacks with persistent visual disturbances (eg, false motion in peripheral vision, color flashes, halos); synesthesia
MDMA	Mydriasis		Esophoria		Blurred	
Rohypnol	Mydriasis; variable pupil size			Injection, watering eyes	Blurred	
Salvia						Altered perceptions of visual stimuli

Data from refs.[1,2]

zombie-like gait, chaotic blindness, confusion, auditory and visual hallucinations, and difficulty recognizing people and objects. At doses higher than 15 mg/kg, delusions, hallucinations, and psychosis occur, and there is perceived blindness and a sense of losing connection with one's body. Tachycardia, hypertension, diaphoresis, mydriasis, nystagmus, slurred speech, and poor motor coordination signal intoxication. A genetically polymorphic enzyme determines a person's ability to metabolize DXM in the liver, so the intensity of DXM effects for any dose is concordantly highly variable. Toxicity can present as severe serotonin syndrome without another serotonergic drug being taken. High-dose chronic DXM use has presented as chronic bromism toxicity with neuromuscular effects and bromoderma acne. Tolerance builds rapidly, dependence has been reported, and withdrawal symptoms include fatigue, apathy, constipation, sleep disturbance, and anxiety. Of particular concern is the cumulative toxicity from using combination DXM preparations, classically high-dose acetaminophen, causing life-threatening hepatotoxicity.

GAMMA-HYDROXYBUTYRATE

Often used as a parachute to come down from an Ecstasy high, GHB is a club drug used for its perceived safe profile of effects, which include euphoria, disinhibition, sedation, and enhanced sexual performance.[1,2,18,19] Owing to its anesthetic properties, GHB is one of the most commonly used date rape drugs. GHB effects start about 10 to 20 minutes after ingestion. Dose-dependent depressant effects last 2 to 6 hours and can result in the classic toxicity triad of coma, bradycardia, and myoclonus. Pathognomonic for GHB is the spontaneous remission of unexplained coma to a normal or hyperalert state. Myoclonic jerking may occur as part the emergence phenomenon from coma. Individuals who regularly use GHB often present with mild-to-moderate symptoms, including anxiety, irritability, mood swings, aggression, insomnia, and hallucinations. Tolerance and dependence can develop quickly.[18] Withdrawal symptoms that occur 1 to 6 hours after last use and last 9 to 14 days resemble those seen with alcohol withdrawal, including nausea, vomiting, diaphoresis, insomnia, restlessness, irritability, anxiety, tremor, and delirium.[18]

INHALANTS

The 3 subgroups of inhalants are volatile solvents, fuels, and anesthetics; nitrous oxide; and volatile alkyl nitrites. The first subgroup is the most popular among youth.[1,2,20,21] The pleasurable sensory high caused by inhalants occurs rapidly and includes effects resembling those of anesthesia, including light-headedness and disinhibition. Continued intake extends initial intoxication from several minutes to several hours, with slurred speech, dizziness, diplopia, disorientation, and ataxia evident at higher doses. Symptoms typically resolve quickly with few hangover effects, although euphoria often leaves a lingering headache and drowsiness. Potential evidence of recent use includes inhalant halitosis, chemical stains or paint on clothes or skin, or face or airway frostbite from aerosol computer cleaners. Huffer rash, a perioral or perinasal eczema with pyoderma can occur with repeated use. Sudden sniffing death syndrome is the primary cause of inhalant use fatality, because with each use the inhalant sensitizes the myocardium in a way that can trigger a fatal cardiac arrhythmia. Inhaling nitrites is associated with men having sex with men, and can cause clinically significant methemoglobinemia. Many pathologic effects of inhalant use reverse when use is stopped, but the lipid-rich nervous system is the most vulnerable to chronic exposure and permanent damage.

Tolerance to and dependence on inhalants can occur, and withdrawal symptoms have been reported.

KETAMINE

Ketamine is a dissociative anesthetic currently used for human and veterinary anesthesia.[1–3,22–24] Dissociative anesthetics do not produce classic hallucinations, but instead lead to perceptual distortions of sound and sight and a sense of detachment or disconnection from one's surroundings and body. Depending on the route of ketamine administration, the effects begin between 2 to 15 minutes later and generally last several hours. A ketamine high, typically called a "trip to K-land," is described as a relaxed, floating feeling of being separated from one's body. An individual using ketamine can seem to be catatonic with rigid posturing and flat facies along with a fixed sightless stare. Hallucinations, visual distortions, and a sense of altered time perception are commonly reported. Higher doses can yield social withdrawal and impaired cognition characterized by bizarre thought patterns and responses. Users "in the K-hole" may show marked motor impairment or true catatonia and report frightening near-death experiences with sensations of loss of time and identity. Repeated and prolonged use can lead to chronic memory impairment, confusion, and "word blocking," as well as development of tolerance and dependence. Because ketamine is odorless, causes amnesia, and can be unknowingly ingested in a beverage, it is used as a date rape drug.

LYSERGIC ACID DIETHYLAMIDE

LSD is a true illusinogenic substance because it induces a perceptual distortion of a real stimulus, whereas an hallucinogenic substance induces perceived sensations that do not exist.[1–3,22,23] Typically ingested orally as sugar cubes or absorbent paper (blotter), LSD's effects start 30 to 90 minutes later and last up to 12 hours. The LSD trip experience depends on the dose, the user's personality, mood, expectations and setting. Pleasant trips involve visual distortions of shapes and movements, and can be mentally stimulating. The main emotional and sensory effects of LSD may manifest in *synesthesia,* a phenomenon that involves intensified and blended sensory perceptions such as "tasting sounds" or "feeling colors." Conversely, a "bad trip" can be an acutely dysphoric experience with thoughts of despair and nightmare-like sensations of doom, anxiety, and panic, or fears of losing control, insanity, or death. Other physiologic responses include tachycardia, dilated pupils, dizziness, anorexia, sweating, nausea, and fine tremor. Tolerance to LSD effects can develop quickly, yet dissipate quickly with abstinence, and physical withdrawal symptoms have not been reported. Two long-term LSD disorders can occur: persistent psychosis, and hallucinogen persisting perceptual disorder, that is, flashbacks. LSD psychosis resembles acute schizophrenic psychosis except that LSD hallucinations are mostly visual, whereas schizophrenic hallucinations are typically auditory. Flashbacks include persistent visual disturbances, for example, false motion in peripheral vision, bright and colorful flashes, and halos or light trails on moving objects. When LSD is ingested together with "other" drugs, they do not interact to cause additive adverse reactions.

METHYLENEDIOXYMETHAMPHETAMINE (ALSO CALLED ECSTASY OR MOLLY)

MDMA is one of the most popular amphetamine analog designer drugs and probably the most well-known club drug.[1–3,11,22,25] Acting on both serotonin and norepinephrine release, MDMA has both psychedelic and stimulant effects. Within 20 to 60 minutes after MDMA ingestion, users experience a sense of general well-being, empathy, emotional warmth and acceptance, decreased anxiety, and mental stimulation, typically lasting 2 to 3 hours. Sensory enhancement and illusory distortions are the hallmark of MDMA intoxication. Owing to its action as a selective serotonin neurotoxin, MDMA also causes muscle ache and the involuntary jaw clenching and bruxism that leads to the popular use of pacifiers in rave settings. Common physical signs of use include mydriasis, tachycardia, and hypertension. When MDMA is paired with extended intense physical activity, such as all-night dancing at raves, potentially serious or fatal dehydration, hyperthermia, rhabdomyolysis, or kidney failure can result. At high doses, arrhythmias, heart failure, hepatic failure, panic attack, and seizures can occur. Because MDMA metabolites block further metabolism, high-dose use can very rapidly cause toxic effects. Ecstasy tablets have been tested on site at raves and found to contain adulterants and "other" psychoactive drugs, including methamphetamine, caffeine, ketamine, or DXM. MDMA users often engage in drug "stacking," that is, combining MDMA with alcohol or marijuana, or they ingest multiple MDMA tablets at once, or intentionally ingest MDMA and LSD concurrently, called "candy flipping." Anxiety, sadness, irritability, and sleepiness can last a week or more after moderate MDMA use. Withdrawal symptoms include fatigue, difficulty concentrating, anorexia, and depression.

FLUNITRAZEPAM (ROHYPNOL)

A benzodiazepine 10 times more potent than diazepam, Rohypnol is a central nervous system depressant with anxiolytic, muscle relaxant, sedative-hypnotic, amnestic, and anticonvulsant effects.[1,2,22] Rohypnol is odorless and tasteless, dissolves readily in carbonated beverages, and produces anterograde amnesia, factors that contribute to its use as a date rape drug. At low doses, Rohypnol produces alcohol-like intoxication with decreased anxiety, muscle relaxation, disinhibition, drowsiness, slurred speech, and psychomotor slowing. Higher doses lead to bradycardia, respiratory depression, confusion, loss of muscle control, loss of consciousness, and amnesia. Onset of effects is within 30 minutes, peaking at 2 hours, and lasting about 8 to 12 hours. Rohypnol is popular among heroin and cocaine users because it potentiates the depressant effects of heroin, and acts as a crash-mitigating "parachute" after cocaine use. As with other benzodiazepines, prolonged use of Rohypnol can lead to tolerance and dependence, plus withdrawal symptoms such as restlessness, anxiety, headache, myalgia, photosensitivity, numbness, and increased seizure potential. Of the drugs discussed in this article, Rohypnol is the only one for which a specific medication, a short-acting benzodiazepine antagonist, can reverse acute intoxication. The standard protocol for treating benzodiazepine withdrawal applies as well.

SALVIA DIVINORUM (SALVIA)

When salvia leaves are dried and smoked or vaporized, the hallucinogenic and dissociative effects begin within 1 minute and last about 30 minutes.[1-3,11,26] Chewing fresh leaves delays onset to about 5 to 10 minutes and effects last 1 to 2 hours. Salvia can produce brief hallucinations mimicking psychosis, and users experience disorientation, feelings of detachment or disembodiment, and sensations of traveling through time and space, floating, flying, or spinning. These altered perceptions of external reality, oneself, and visual stimuli can result in difficulty interacting safely with one's surroundings. Many users decline trying salvia more than once and its popularity is waning.

SYNTHETIC CANNABINOIDS

This category includes a large number of unregulated compounds that mimic the structure of tetrahydrocannabinoid (the psychoactive chemical in marijuana) and are marketed as legal marijuana alternatives.[1–2,25–27] Users start feeling relaxed and sleepy with an elevated mood and altered sense of reality about 4 to 5 minutes after smoking, and the effects last from 1 to 8 hours. Synthetic cannabinoids bind to the same receptors as tetrahydrocannabinoid, but are 4 to 10 times more potent and can produce unpredictable effects, including chest pain, paranoia, delusions, and hallucinations. Other adverse effects include tachycardia, hypertension, vomiting, confusion, and agitation. The plethora of ever-changing products being designed may contain no actual cannabinoids, or unknown products more dangerous than tetrahydrocannabinoid. Symptoms of overdose include seizures, myocardial ischemia, anxiety attack, and stroke. Although dependence and withdrawal have been reported, long-term effects of synthetic cannabinoid use remain unknown.

SYNTHETIC CATHINONES (BATH SALTS)

These refer to a family of substances including 3,4 methylenedioxypyrovalerone, mephedrone and methylone, among others, that are analogs to cathinone, the active ingredient found in Khat shrub leaves that are chewed in some African and Asian cultures for their stimulant effects.[1,2,19,25,26,28] Bath salts, advertised for bathing, plant food, or other uses, are manufactured solely for substance abuse purposes. These central nervous system stimulants cause feelings of agitation and increased energy within 15 minutes of ingestion, and lead to 4 to 6 hours of effects that include alertness, talkativeness, sociability, and intense euphoria. Higher doses cause perceptual distortions, diaphoresis, emesis, tachycardia, hypertension, hyperthermia, headache, and seizures, and can result in altered mental status with paranoia, delusions, hallucinations, and violent behavior, including self-mutilation and suicidal or homicidal activity. Chronic users can develop tolerance and dependence, so that withdrawal symptoms, including craving, chills, sweats, and hallucinations, may be severe enough to require medical supervision.

SUMMARY

Adolescents who engage in risk-taking behaviors, including early use of gateway nicotine, alcohol, or marijuana, and those experiencing academic or psychosocial problems are more likely to engage in or already be engaged in substance use, including club drugs, hallucinogens, and inhalants. Despite decreases in use by adolescents, the club drugs and "other" drugs discussed in this article will remain among the evolving selection of substances used. Adolescents most often use the least expensive, most accessible substances they perceive to have the lowest risks, which can describe club drugs and "other" drugs, such as inhalants. The simultaneous use of multiple and unknown substances is common among adolescents, often as an unintended consequence of substances being contaminated, adulterated or substituted in composition, known to occur commonly with club drugs and designer drugs. Polysubstance use causes mixed and variable effects, patient experiences and patient presentations, particularly to an acute or emergency care setting. Physicians working in emergency settings are most likely to provide care to substance-using patients who are 'high' or experiencing adverse effects, and in the case of this article's drugs, eye findings and vision changes can often provide important diagnostic clues. Multiple drug use should always be considered whenever any drug use is suspected or detected. Most of the substances discussed in this article cannot be detected by routine urine toxicology screens, so it is useful for health care providers to be familiar with local laboratory drug testing panels, protocols, and limitations. All providers should be alert for potentially more subtle telltale behaviors, signs, symptoms, and symbols or paraphernalia indicative of or associated with substance use. For club drug use, this includes use of pacifiers, menthol inhalers, and surgical masks.

The risk of sudden death and the generally younger age of inhalant users should serve to remind health care practitioners to screen for inhalant use when caring for young adolescents, male patients having sex with men, and patients with occupational inhalant exposure or availability. To facilitate all levels of substance use-related patient care from prevention and SBIRT practices to substance use detection and emergency management, it is most helpful for providers to be aware of current local and regional substance use trends, specific use-related acute and chronic health effects, and any available care and referral resources.

REFERENCES

1. Williams J, Lundahl LH, Fortune RSD. Evolving array of substances used by adolescents. Adolesc Med 2014;025:184–214.
2. National Institute on Drug Abuse. Drugs of abuse. 2019. Available at: https://www.drugabuse.gov/drugs-abuse. Accessed July 15, 2019.
3. MacLean KA, Johnson MW, Griffiths RR. Hallucinogens and club drugs. In: Galanter M, Kleber HD, Brady KT, editors. The American psychiatric publishing textbook of substance abuse treatment. 5th edition. Arlington (VA): American Psychiatric Publishing; 2015. p. 209–22.
4. Johnston LD, Miech RA, O'Malley PM, et al. Monitoring the Future national survey results on drug use, 1975-2018: overview, key findings on adolescent drug use. Ann Arbor: Institute for Social Research, University of Michigan. Available at: http://www.monitoringthefuture.org/. Accessed March 1, 2019.
5. Miech RA, Johnston LD, O'Malley PM, et al. Monitoring the Future national survey results on drug use, 1975–2018: volume I, Secondary school students. Ann Arbor (MI): Institute for Social Research, The University of Michigan; 2019. Available at: http://monitoringthefuture.org/pubs.html#monographs.
6. Schulenberg JE, Johnston LD, O'Malley PM, et al. Monitoring the Future national survey results on drug use, 1975–2018: volume II, College students and adults ages 19–60. Ann Arbor (MI): Institute for Social Research, The University of Michigan; 2019. Available at: http://monitoringthefuture.org/pubs.html#monographs.
7. Johnston LD, Miech RA, O'Malley PM, et al. Demographic subgroup trends among adolescents in the use of various licit and illicit drugs, 1975–2018 (Monitoring the Future Occasional Paper No. 92). Ann Arbor (MI): Institute for Social Research, The University of Michigan; 2019.
8. Substance Abuse and Mental Health Services Administration. Key substance use and mental health indicators in the United States: results from the 2016 national survey on drug use and health (HHS publication No. SMA 17-5044, NSDUH series H-52). Rockville (MD): Center for Behavioral Health Statistics and Quality, Substance Abuse and Mental Health Services Administration; 2017. Available at: https://www.samhsa.gov/data/.

9. U.S. Department of Justice. Drug enforcement administration. Diversion control division. Drug and chemical information. Available at: https://www.deadiversion. usdoj.gov/drug_chem_info/index.html. Accessed July 15, 2019.

10. DEA intelligence report (unclassified). Slang terms and code words: a reference for law enforcement personnel. DEA-HOU-DIR-022-18. Available at: https://www. drugabuse.gov/drugs-abuse. Accessed June19, 2019.

11. Erowid. Psychoactive plants and drugs. 2019. Available at: https://erowid.org/ psychoactives/. Accessed June19, 2019.

12. AAP Committee on Substance Use and Prevention. Substance use screening, brief intervention, and referral to treatment. Pediatrics 2016;138(1):e20161210.

13. Levy SJ, Williams JF, AAP Committee on Substance Use and Prevention. Substance use screening, brief intervention, and referral to treatment. Pediatrics 2016;138(1):e20161211.

14. Kwong T, Magnani B, Rosano T, et al, editors. The clinical toxicology laboratory: contemporary practice of poisoning evaluation. 2nd edition. Washington, DC: AACC Press; 2013.

15. Levy S, Siqueira LM, AAP Committee on Substance Use and Prevention. Testing for drugs of abuse in children and adolescents. Pediatrics 2014;133:e1798.

16. Williams JF, Kokotailo PK. Abuse of proprietary (over-the-counter) drugs. Adolesc Med Clin 2006;17(3):733–50.

17. Boyer EW. Dextromethophan abuse. Pediatr Emerg Care 2004;20(12):858–63.

18. McDonough M, Kennedy N, Glasper A, et al. Clinical features and management of gamma-hydroxybutyrate (GHB) withdrawal: a review. Drug Alcohol Depend 2004;75(1):3–9.

19. Karila L, Reynaud M. GHB and synthetic cathinones: clinical effects and potential consequences. Drug Test Anal 2011;3(9):552–9.

20. NIH National Institute on Drug Abuse. Inhalants. Research Report Series: NIH publication number 12-3818. Revised July 2012. Available at: https:// d14rmgtrwzf5a.cloudfront.net/sites/default/files/inhalantsrrs.pdf.

21. Wu LT, Schlenger WE, Ringwalt CL. Use of nitrite inhalants ("poppers") among American youth. J Adolesc Health 2005;37(1):52–60.

22. Rome ES. It's a rave new world: rave culture and illicit drug use in the young. Cleve Clin J Med 2001;68(6):541–50.

23. National Institute on Drug Abuse. DrugFacts: hallucinogens – LSD, Peyote, Psilocybin, and PCP. Available at: http://www.drugabuse.gov/publications/drugfacts/ hallucinogens-lsd-peyote-psilocybin-pcp. Accessed November 20, 2018..

24. Morgan CJ, Curran HV. Independent scientific committee on drugs. Ketamine use: a review. Addiction 2012;107(1):27–38.

25. Klega AE, Keehbauch JT. Stimulant and designer drug use: primary care management. Am Fam Physician 2018;98(2):85–92.

26. Rosenbaum CD, Carreiro SP, Babu KM. Here today, gone tomorrow...and back again? A review of herbal marijuana alternatives (K2, Spice), synthetic cathinones (bath salts), kratom, Salvia divinorum, methoxetamine, and piperazines. J Med Toxicol 2012;8(1):15–32.

27. National Institute on Drug Abuse. DrugFacts: spice (synthetic marijuana) 2012. Available at: http://www.drugabuse.gov/publications/drugfacts/spice-synthetic-marijuana. Accessed November 12, 2018.

28. Prosser JM, Nelson LS. The toxicology of bath salts: a review of synthetic cathinones. J Med Toxicol 2012;8(1):33–42.

Cocaine Use in Adolescents and Young Adults

Sheryl A. Ryan, MD*

KEYWORDS

- Cocaine • Crack cocaine • Cocaine use disorder • Neurobiology • Withdrawal
- Adolescents • Young adults

KEY POINTS

- Cocaine use, although less common than alcohol, tobacco, or marijuana use, continues to be used by significant numbers of adolescents and young adults.
- Cocaine is a potent stimulant with central nervous system effects through its ability to increase levels of neurotransmitters such as dopamine, norepinephrine and serotonin.
- Long-term heavy use of cocaine poses significant health effects on many organ systems mainly through its stimulation of the sympathetic nervous system.
- Diagnostic and Statistical Manual of Mental Disorders Fifth Edition criteria are used to determine whether individuals meet criteria of mild, moderate, or severe cocaine use disorders.
- Because there are no Food and Drug Administration–approved agents to treat cocaine use disorders, behavioral therapies are the mainstay of treatment.

INTRODUCTION

Cocaine has been estimated to be second only to heroin according to ranking scores that have used evidence-based data to assess drug "harmfulness."[1] Cocaine is a tropane ester alkaloid made from the leaves of the Erythroxylum coca plant, a bush that is native to the Andes Mountain regions of South America (chiefly Colombia, Peru, and Bolivia). It is an addictive stimulant drug and is used in 2 main forms: powder cocaine and crack. Common street names for cocaine and crack include snow, rock, flake, toot, candy, line, and blow.

Magnitude of Use by Adolescents and Young Adults

According to the Monitoring the Future study, in 2017, 2.7% of 12th graders reported annual use of cocaine, and 0.5% reported annual use of crack cocaine; 1.4% and

Disclosure Statement: The author has no financial conflicts to disclose.
Division of Adolescent Medicine, Department of Pediatrics, Milton S. Hershey Medical Center, Penn State Hershey Children's Hospital, Hershey, PA 17033, USA
* 500 University Drive, Hershey, PA 17033.
E-mail address: Sryan4@pennstatehealth.psu.edu

Pediatr Clin N Am 66 (2019) 1135–1147
https://doi.org/10.1016/j.pcl.2019.08.014
0031-3955/19/© 2019 Elsevier Inc. All rights reserved.

pediatric.theclinics.com

0.6% of 10th graders and 0.8% and 1.0% of 8th graders reported annual use of cocaine and crack cocaine, respectively.[2] Results from the 2017 National Survey of Drug Use and Health[3] indicate that an estimated 0.1% of 12 to 17 year olds (about 26,000 individuals) and 1.9% of 18 to 25 year olds (about 665,000 individuals) reported current cocaine (including crack cocaine) use. Significantly higher numbers of 18 to 25 year olds reported past-year rates than adolescents aged 12 to 17 years: 6.2% and 0.3% of 18 to 25 year olds reported past-year use of cocaine and crack cocaine, respectively, compared with 0.5% and 0.1% of 12 to 17 year olds. Finally, in 2017, 0.1% of the 12 to 17-year-old population and 0.7% of 18 to 25 year olds met Diagnostic and Statistical Manual of Mental Disorders Fourth Edition[3] criteria for a cocaine use disorder.[4]

Although peak ages for cocaine dependence are between 23 and 25 years of age, once use begins, cocaine dependence develops far more rapidly and "explosively" than what is seen with either marijuana or alcohol. For example, up to 5% to 6% of cocaine users will develop dependence within the first year of use.[5] Cocaine use is also highly associated with the use of other licit and illicit substances, and comorbid psychiatric conditions such as anxiety and depression.[6] Further, the earlier an adolescent begins using an illicit substance, including cocaine, the higher the risk of developing problems related to that use.[7]

EPIDEMIOLOGY

Cocaine use occurs among all demographic and socioeconomic groups.[4] Among those aged 12 to 17 years, past-year cocaine use was higher among Caucasians (0.6%), Latinos (0.5%), and those reporting 2 or more races (0.9%) compared with Blacks (0.1%), Native or Alaskan Americans (0.2%), or Asians (0.3%). For young adults aged 18 to 25 years, highest rates of past-year use were reported by Native/Alaskan Americans (10.6%) and those reporting 2 or more races (9.2%), followed by Caucasians (7.6%) and Latinos (6.2%), with Blacks (1.9%) and Asians (2.0%) reporting the lowest rates. For youth 12 to 17 years of age, no gender differences were seen with reported past-year use of cocaine; however, for 18 to 25 year olds, men reported higher rates than women. Results of the few studies investigating factors contributing to the use of cocaine by adolescents and young adults have found correlations between early onset of substance use and childhood history of behavioral, conduct, or antisocial behaviors, association with "deviant" peers, inadequate parental monitoring or supervision, and parental use of illicit substances.[8] Conversely, protective factors include role modeling of nonparent adults, development of social skills, participation in recreational activities, and religiosity.[9]

PHARMACOLOGY OF COCAINE

During the process of extraction of cocaine from the coca plant leaves, 2 forms are produced: a base form and a salt form. The base form is created by heating the salt form in an organic solvent that has a base pH, a process also knows as "free-basing" with the resulting formation of crack cocaine. This has a low melting point (98° C) and vaporizes readily before destruction of the active compound occurs. As a result, it can be smoked but cannot be injected because of its insolubility in water. In contrast, the salt form of cocaine, a white powder, cannot be smoked because it melts at a much higher temperature than the base form (195° C) and is destroyed before it vaporizes. However, it is readily injected or "snorted" through nasal mucosa and is highly water soluble, allowing for it to be easily dissolved and injected. Cocaine is readily absorbed through oral and nasal mucous membrane as well as from the respiratory, gastrointestinal, genitourinary tracts. Following ingestion, it is rapidly distributed and taken up into most organs including the brain, heart, kidney, adrenal glands, and liver. It can also be measured in blood, urine, hair, sweat, and breast milk; analysis of these fluids and tissues can be used for detection for legal, workplace, or treatment purposes.

The average purity of the salt form of cocaine powder is about 50%, and a variety of additives or adulterants are mixed with the powder. These additives can be inert and include lactose, dextrose, or starch, or active, such as benzocaine, procaine, hydroxyzine, diltiazem, phenacetin, or lidocaine. Psychoactive adulterants such as amphetamines, caffeine, phencyclidine, or ephedrine have been used and can potentially enhance or complicate the effects.

When cocaine is inhaled by smoking, or through injection, the onset and maximal peak effect occurs within minutes, and lasts for 15 to 30 minutes. When snorted intranasally, onset of action is slower, occurring within 30 to 45 minutes, with a longer peak effect and a more gradual decline to baseline—more than 60 to 90 minutes.[10]

Once ingested, cocaine undergoes metabolism via both liver and serum cholinesterases to 2 main metabolites, benzoylecgonine and ecgonine methyl ester. These substances are water soluble and readily excreted in the urine. The serum half-life of cocaine is between 45 and 90 minutes; thus, cocaine can be measured in either serum or urine only for several hours after ingestion. The metabolites can be detected in blood and urine up to 24 to 36 hours after use and toxicologic tests measuring the metabolites of benzoylecgonine and ecgonine provide evidence of recent use.[11]

MECHANISMS OF ACTION OF COCAINE IN THE CENTRAL AND PERIPHERAL NERVOUS SYSTEMS

The central neural circuit that has been the most studied and implicated in explaining the psychotropic and reinforcing effects of many addictive substances, including cocaine, is the mesocorticolimbic dopaminergic system.[12] This circuit includes brain structures integral for reward processing, impulse control, and inhibition[13]; it consists of dopaminergic cells in the ventral tegmental area located in the mesencephalon that project to structures in the forebrain such as the nucleus accumbens and the prefrontal cortex (**Fig. 1**). Studies using functional MRI (fMRI), PET, and single-photon emission computed tomography techniques have found that these brain regions show increased blood flow or activity in response to stimulants such as cocaine.[14]

Cocaine is similar to all stimulants in that it increases the extracellular and synaptic levels of monoamine neurotransmitters, such as dopamine, norepinephrine, and serotonin, which are integral to the normal functioning of the mesocorticolimbic circuit. Binding to the monoamine transporters located at nerve endings, dendrites, axons, and cell bodies, it blocks the reuptake of released monoamine neurotransmitters into neuronal cells. As a result, levels of synaptic dopamine are increased well above levels that are normally experienced through natural rewards, resulting in the acute euphoric effect experienced by cocaine users. This effect of cocaine on the reward circuit systems of the brain also lends support to observed difficulties with impulse control and cravings seen with cocaine use.[15] Several psychiatric disorders such as depression, anxiety, attention

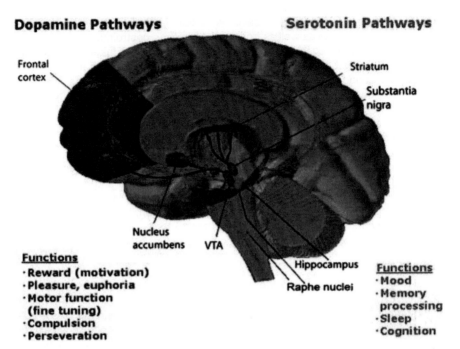

Dopamine Pathways   **Serotonin Pathways**

Frontal cortex

Striatum

Substantia nigra

Nucleus accumbens   VTA

Hippocampus

Raphe nuclei

Functions
- **Reward (motivation)**
- **Pleasure, euphoria**
- **Motor function (fine tuning)**
- **Compulsion**
- **Perseveration**

Functions
- **Mood**
- **Memory processing**
- **Sleep**
- **Cognition**

Fig. 1. Dopamine and serotonin pathways and functions. (*From* Deter, DT. Understanding the Disease of Addiction. Primary Care Clinics 38(1):1-7, DOI: 10.1016/j.pop.2010.11.001 with permission.)

deficit disorder, and schizophrenia have been found to be associated with dysfunction of this system.

CLINICAL MANIFESTATIONS
Acute Intoxication

The initial desired effect of cocaine use is euphoria. In addition, those using cocaine will experience increased energy, alertness, and sociability and decreased appetite and need for sleep. With increased duration of use, higher doses, or more efficient routes of administration, individuals may experience dysphoric effects such as anxiety, irritability, restlessness, and agitation; these may be especially prominent when the individual is coming down from a "high." Up to 30% of cocaine users report symptoms that include anxiety, depression, sleep problems, and weight loss.[16] **Table 1** lists the signs and symptoms commonly seen with acute intoxication, and **Table 2** lists adverse effects experienced with higher doses and more efficient methods of ingesting cocaine, such as through inhalation or intravenously.

Psychotic symptoms resembling acute schizophrenia can be experienced with higher doses and longer duration of use. Younger age is an independent risk factor for developing psychotic symptoms.[17] Compared with acute schizophrenia, patients with a cocaine use disorder may report more paranoia but fewer disordered thoughts and delusions. They may experience both auditory and tactile hallucinations, with fewer being visual.[18] A prominent tactile hallucination is formication or the sense of insects or parasites crawling under one's skin.

Table 1
Signs and symptoms of acute cocaine intoxication

Symptoms	Signs
Euphoria—"Cocaine high"	Increased blood pressure
Intense pleasurable feelings	Elevated heart rate
Increased energy	Dilated pupils—mydriasis
Increased sociability	Diaphoresis
Decreased fatigue	Nausea/vomiting
Decreased need for sleep	Hyperventilation
Decreased appetite	Tremor
Restlessness	Acute coronary syndrome
	Seizures
	Rhabdomyolysis
	Hyperthermia
	Stroke

EFFECTS OF COCAINE ON SPECIFIC ORGAN SYSTEMS

With long-term and heavy use of cocaine, widespread and potentially lethal effects are seen throughout many organ systems. Many of these systemic effects result from the direct effect of cocaine's heightened stimulation of the sympathetic nervous system, causing peripheral vasoconstriction and organ ischemia. These effects can also be seen during intoxication or with first-time users.

Central Nervous System

Central nervous system effects include strokes, seizures, and movement disorders. A 5.7-fold increase in the risk of ischemic stroke was seen in a group of 15 to 49 year olds, even after adjusting for stroke risk factors such as tobacco use. In those reporting use immediately before the stroke, the greatest risk was within 6 hours of the reported cocaine use. It has been postulated that acute increases in blood pressure have contributed to the increased incidence in hemorrhagic types of stroke.[19]

Generalized, tonic-clonic, and partial seizures can be seen with first-time use and without any prior reports of seizure disorders. Most of these occur within the initial 60 minutes after ingestion when peak plasma concentrations are reached. These seizures are generally single, and do not require medication for control, although status epilepticus and repeat seizures have been reported.[20]

Table 2
Adverse psychological and behavioral effects of chronic cocaine use

Psychological	Behavioral
Anxiety, panic attacks	Agitation
Irritability	Restlessness
Dysphoria	Tremors
Paranoia	Dyskinesia
Hypervigilance	Stereotypical behaviors (ie, picking at skin)
Grandiosity	Impaired judgment
Psychotic symptoms	May result in involvement in high-risk behavior
Hallucinations—visual and tactile	

Cardiac

Cardiac symptoms are the most common symptoms reported by those seeking medical care as a result of their cocaine use, with chest pain being the most frequent complaint. Through its combined effects of being a powerful sympathomimetic agent and through its adrenergic effects, it can acutely increase blood pressure, heart rate, and peripheral vascular resistance and stimulate coronary artery alpha-adrenergic receptors. The result may be coronary artery vasoconstriction with potential acute myocardial ischemia (MI) and/or infarction. The highest risk for ischemia is during the first 60 minutes after use, even in young individuals with no prior risk factors or small vessel disease,[21] and is independent of the amount used, the route of ingestion, or the frequency of use.[22] Cocaine use has been reported as the leading cause of death among young adults using illicit substances[23] and has been reported as a factor in 25% of nonfatal MIs in people younger than 45 years.[24] Long-term side effects on cardiac function are uncommon but have been reported.

Respiratory System

The respiratory effects of cocaine use are more likely to be seen with those who smoke and inhale crack cocaine. Fifty percent of users who smoke cocaine will experience acute shortness of breath, cough, wheezing, or hemoptysis; asthma exacerbation can also be seen.[25,26] When cocaine is insufflated (sniffed), both acute and chronic effects can be seen in the nasal and oral cavities.[27]

Renal System

Acute renal failure secondary to rhabdomyolysis can occur with acute cocaine use.[28]

Psychological and Cognitive Function

Several studies have reported that long-term cocaine use results in significant adverse effects on cognition, specifically in the areas of executive processing, attention, and working memory, and on social functioning and interactions.[29] In a recent systematic critical review of cognitive and neuroimaging studies done between 1999 and 2016 (N = 47) in cocaine users, Frazer and colleagues[30] found that "the current evidence does not support the view that chronic cocaine use is associated with broad cognitive deficits." They found no consistency among fMRI and imaging studies assessing the role of acute and chronic cocaine use on structural white or gray matter changes in brains of adults using cocaine and concluded that "converging evidence suggests that the compensatory neuroplastic changes associated with chronic cocaine exposure likely create conditions where cognitive performance is normalized during acute intoxication, declines during withdrawal, and recovers gradually over the course of abstinence".[30]

MANAGEMENT OF ACUTE INTOXICATION

When a teen or young adult presents to the emergency room with a constellation of symptoms that suggest acute intoxication (see **Table 1**), cocaine use should be considered, along with the use of other licit and illicit substances. It is also important to rule out other possible causes that may present similarly, such as hyperthyroidism, hypoglycemia, or psychiatric disorders such as panic attacks, mania from bipolar disorder, or acute schizophrenia. Toxicologic screens of both urine and blood are important, although it must be noted that blood concentrations are often not helpful prognostically, given that the blood concentrations generally do not correlate well with severity of symptoms.[31]

Initial management of acute intoxication presenting in the emergency department should be nonpharmacologic and focus on providing a safe and quiet environment for the teen or young adult, with as little stimulation as possible. Restraints should be avoided. The 2 major potential complications that need to be considered and are mentioned earlier include seizures and acute chest pain that may indicate cardiac ischemia. Both of these can be seen within the first hours of use, during acute ingestion and intoxication. The reader is referred to a comprehensive discussion of the management of cardiac complications.[32]

WITHDRAWAL

Hospitalization is rarely needed for medical reasons in those adolescents or young adults experiencing withdrawal, given that physical symptoms are less prominent than psychological symptoms and rarely life threatening. The individual may experience mild and transient nonspecific musculoskeletal pain or discomfort, chills, tremors, or involuntary muscle movements. MI has been reported to occur in the first week of withdrawal. Thus, any individual presenting during this time with chest pain or symptoms that suggest MI should be urgently evaluated.[32]

The psychological symptoms of withdrawal are more common and problematic. These include depression, anxiety, fatigue, difficulty concentrating, anhedonia, craving, increased appetite, and increased need for sleep.[10] In some cases, the depression and psychomotor retardation can be severe and debilitating and may be associated with suicidal ideation and attempts. Currently, there are no medications that have been found to be effective or approved specifically for cocaine withdrawal.

EVALUATION AND DIAGNOSIS OF COCAINE USE DISORDERS
Assessment/Screening

Several well-validated screening tools can be used with adolescents and young adults, such as the CRAFFT,[33] the S2BI,[34] and the 2-question National Institute on Alcohol Abuse and Alcoholism screener.[35] These generally identify whether there is any use of alcohol or drugs such as cocaine, for example, that warrants further investigation. Ask the teen or young adult directly about when the cocaine use started, how frequently it is used, whether this use has escalated, specific pattern of use, and methods of use. Asking about the use of other substances such as alcohol, tobacco, marijuana, or prescription opioids or stimulants is important, as cocaine use is most likely preceded by use of other substances. The provider should inquire about involvement in high-risk behaviors that may be linked to episodes of intoxication, such as driving while intoxicated or interpersonal violence. Unsafe sexual practices or the sharing of needles with injected substances can result in the acquisition of infections such as hepatitis B, C, or human immunodeficiency virus (HIV). Also query past or current history of medical and psychiatric conditions and treatment, family history of substance use/abuse, and psychiatric disorders and conduct a review of systems and complete psychosocial and developmental history.

A structured interview tool such as the HEEADSSS[36] screener allows assessment of social functioning and development in the areas of school or work, the home environment, and relationships with friends and family members. Noting both strengths as well as deficits is essential. Because the onset of significant substance use and abuse has been identified as a factor in the derailment of normative adolescent development,[37] it is important to identify whether the adolescent or young adult is achieving age-appropriate developmental milestones. Questions about progression through school, identification and progress toward future career, job, or life goals and demonstrated autonomy and responsibility for one's health and welfare are all important. A full review of all organ systems and mental health symptoms will identify whether the cocaine use or the concomitant use of other substances has caused any medical complications.

A full physical examination, focusing on vital signs and key organ systems such as the cardiac, pulmonary, and neurologic systems needs to be done. Looking for any stigmata of cocaine use, such as nasal irritation, oral lesions, or skin lesions secondary to injection should be included. A mental status examination can provide information about the youth's motivation around treatment as well as orientation, attention span, cognitive capacity, and mood. Laboratory tests can be guided by the information obtained through the history and the physical examination. These may include urine or blood toxicology tests, electrocardiogram, blood chemistries, or tests for sexually transmitted or blood-borne infections such as hepatitis B and C, HIV, Chlamydia trachomatis, and gonorrhea.

Outside of the emergency setting, urine testing for cocaine metabolites is limited because it provides information only about the most recent cocaine use and not about the onset of the substance use, recent pattern of use, or changes over time. These are all obtained through careful and nonjudgmental history taking with the youth in a confidential setting. Conversely, random urine testing can be helpful in monitoring adherence and abstinence during treatment.

At the completion of this initial assessment, a provider should be in a position to identify the extent of the youth's use of cocaine and other substances, the presence of concomitant mental health issues, and medical or psychosocial consequences of the cocaine use. The provider may determine that the teen or young adult has symptoms that indicate a cocaine use disorder or may determine that further evaluation is needed to confirm this diagnosis. With low levels of use, the provider may elect to do brief intervention in the office setting, using Screening, Brief Intervention, and Referral Treatment approaches.[38] The provider may also determine that the youth needs further assessment or referral for a higher level of care.

TREATMENT STRATEGIES FOR COCAINE USE AND ABUSE

The goals of treatment of any youth using cocaine, regardless of severity, should be complete abstinence of cocaine use. Given the strong cravings that may accompany cocaine use, and the high potential for medical consequences, there can be no support for "controlled use."[39] Additional goals for treatment should include abstinence from the use of any other licit or illicit substances; reduction in substance-associated high-risk behaviors; improvement in social functioning; and progress toward health, well-being, and age-appropriate developmental milestones. A substance use disorder is a chronic recurring disorder that requires continuing care, with expectations for periodic relapses during treatment that may require increasing the intensity of treatment. When resistance is seen during treatment, this may indicate the need to intensify or modify the treatment being provided.

A prominent hallmark that distinguishes cocaine use from other substance use is denial, given the highly reinforcing effect of the euphoria experienced with cocaine.[39] This results often in resistance to accepting the need for and referral to treatment and may also explain the high rates of relapse seen with cocaine use disorders.

In determining the most appropriate level of care that may be required, it is reasonable to start with individual or group outpatient sessions, when it has been determined that the youth has either cocaine use or mild cocaine use disorder. If the youth cannot adhere to treatment recommendations, or when there is a moderate cocaine use disorder, referral to an intensive outpatient program, augmented by either family-based therapy or contingency management components may be necessary. If there is continued inability to comply with recommendations, significant relapse, or a severe cocaine use disorder, residential treatment may be necessary. Unfortunately, in many communities treatment resources for youth with substance use disorders are limited, and this can pose significant barriers to accessing needed treatment. Evidence of this is the fact that juvenile justice programs, and not private or public insurers, are now the largest third-party payers for drug treatment programs for youth in the United States.[40]

Pharmacologic Therapy

There are currently no Food and Drug Administration–approved pharmacologic agents for the treatment of cocaine use disorders. Several experimental approaches are being studied, such as the use of Adderall, or the combination of naltrexone and bupropion, but these are strictly in the experimental stages. When an adolescent or young adult presents with a mental health disorder as well as a substance use disorder, it has been generally recommended that the disorder presenting the most problems for the youth be addressed initially and then the second disorder be addressed. However, there are those who also advocate for treating the substance use disorder initially, as this will enhance the youth's ability to engage in therapy aimed at the psychiatric disorder, such as depression, anxiety, or attention deficit disorder/attention-deficit hyperactivity disorder.

Behavioral Treatment Programs

Behavioral approaches are currently the mainstay of treatment of both cocaine use and cocaine use disorders, although very limited research has been done to evaluate the effectiveness of programs for the treatment of problematic stimulant use, including cocaine. Those that are available have been adapted from those developed

---

Box 1
Behavioral treatment approaches for cocaine use disorders

Brief Interventions

Motivational interviewing[41]

Motivational enhancement therapy (METV)[42]

Cognitive Behavioral Therapy (CBT)[43,44]

Cognitive behavioral therapy with MET component[45]

Contingency Management

Voucher-based reinforcement therapy (VBRT)[46–49]

Family-Based Programs[42,50,51]

Multidimensional family therapy

Multisystemic family therapy

Functional family therapy

Family behavioral therapy
   Family behavioral therapy with MET/CBT component

Brief strategic family therapy

Adolescent community reinforcement approach (ACRA)

specifically for tobacco and alcohol use. These include motivational interviewing, cognitive behavioral therapy programs, contingency management, and family-based treatment programs. Family-based programs have common elements that address parenting skills and family restructuring, such as positive communication, parental monitoring, and supervision, providing positive reinforcement and clear conse-quences tied to negative behaviors and clarifying expectations for substance-related behaviors. **Box 1** lists these and related references. Various types of individual- and group-oriented drug counseling have also been used. Many of these are grounded in the 12-step philosophy but may include cognitive, behavioral, insight-oriented, or supportive approaches.

SUMMARY

Cocaine use remains a significant public health problem for both adolescents and emerging adults. Its use and abuse can cause a wide range of significant medical and psychosocial effects and can disrupt normal psychosocial and psychological development. An understanding of the neurobiology of cocaine provides evidence for its acute intoxication effects as well as long-term physical effects. Few studies have focused on the treatment of cocaine use disorders, although behavioral tech-niques remain the mainstay of treatment. Further research needs to be done to pro-vide information on better options for treatment and their effectiveness.

REFERENCES

1. Nutt D, King LA, Saulsbury W, et al. Development of a rational scale to assess the harm of drugs of potential misuse. Lancet 2007;369(9566):1047–53.
2. Johnston LD, Miech RA, O'Malley PM, et al. Monitoring the future national survey results on drug use: 1975-2017: overview, key findings on adolescent drug use. Ann Arbor (MI): Institute for Social Research, The University of Michigan; 2018. Available at: www.monitoringthefuture.org//pubs/monographs/mtf-overview2017.pdf. Accessed January 26, 2019.
3. American Psychiatric Association. Diagnostic and statistical manual of mental disorders, fifth edition. Arlington (VA): American Psychiatric Association; 2013.
4. Substance Abuse and Mental Health Services Administration. Key substance use and mental health indicators in the United States: results from the 2017 national survey on drug use and health. Rockville (MD): Center for Behavioral Health Sta-tistics and Quality, Substance Abuse and Mental Health Services Administration; 2018 (HHS Publication No. SMA 18-5068, NSDUH Series H-53). Available at: https://www.samhsa.gov/data/.
5. Wagner FA, Anthony JC. From first drug use to drug dependence: developmental periods of risk for dependence upon marijuana, cocaine, and alcohol. Neuropsy-chopharmacology 2002;26(4):479–88.
6. Kandel DB, Huang FY, Davies M. Comorbidity between patterns of substance use dependence and psychiatric syndromes. Drug Alcohol Depend 2001; 64(2):233–41.
7. Anthony JC, Petronis KR. Early-onset drug use and risk of later drug problems. Drug Alcohol Depend 1995;40(1):9–15.
8. Chilcoat HD, Dishion TJ, Anthony JC. Parent monitoring and the incidence of drug sampling in urban elementary school children. Am J Epidemiol 1995; 141(1):25–31.
9. Latimer W, Zur J. Epidemiologic trends of adolescent use of alcohol, tobacco, and other drugs. Child Adolesc Psychiatr Clin N Am 2010;19(3):451–64.

10. Wilkins JN, Danovitch I, Gorelick DA. Management of stimulant, hallucinogen, marijuana, phencyclidine, and club drug intoxication and withdrawal. In: Ries RK, Fiellin DA, Miller SC, et al, editors. The ASAM principles of addiction medicine. Philadelphia: Wolters Kluwer; 2014. p. 685–709.

11. Jeffcoat AR, Perez-Reyes M, Hill JM, et al. Cocaine disposition in humans after intravenous injection, nasal insufflation (snorting), or smoking. Drug Metab Dispos 1989;17(2):153–9.

12. Koob GF. Drugs of abuse: anatomy, pharmacology and function of reward pathways. Trends Pharmacol Sci 1992;13:177–84.

13. Volkow ND, Koob GF, McLellan AT. Neurobiologic advances from the brain disease model of addiction. N Engl J Med 2016;374(4):363–71.

14. Kalivas PW. Neurobiology of cocaine addiction: implications for new pharmacotherapy. Am J Addict 2007;16(2):71–8.

15. Volkow ND, Wang GJ, Fowler JS, et al. Addiction: beyond dopamine reward circuitry. Proc Natl Acad Sci U S A 2011;108(37):15037–42.

16. Williamson S, Gossop M, Powis B, et al. Adverse effects of stimulant drugs in a community sample of drug users. Drug Alcohol Depend 1997;44(2–3):87–94.

17. Smith MJ, Thirthalli J, Abdallah AB, et al. Prevalence of psychotic symptoms in substance users: a comparison across substances. Compr Psychiatry 2009; 50(3):245–50.

18. Roncero C, Ros-Cucurull E, Daigre C, et al. Prevalence and risk factors of psychotic symptoms in cocaine dependent patients. Actas Esp Psiquiatr 2012; 40(4):187–97.

19. Toosi S, Hess CP, Hills NK, et al. Neurovascular complications of cocaine use at a tertiary stroke center. J Stroke Cerebrovasc Dis 2010;19(4):273–8.

20. Neiman J, Haapaniemi HM, Hillbom M. Neurological complications of drug abuse: pathophysiological mechanisms. Eur J Neurol 2000;7(6):595–606.

21. Mittleman MA, Mintzer D, Maclure M, et al. Triggering of myocardial infarction by cocaine. Circulation 1999;99(21):2737–41.

22. Lange RA, Hillis LD. Cardiovascular complications of cocaine use. N Engl J Med 2001;345(5):351–8.

23. Substance Abuse and Mental Health Services Administration. Drug Abuse Warning Network, 2011: National Estimates of Drug-Related Emergency Department Visits. Rockville (MD): Substance Abuse and Mental Health Services Administration; 2013. HHS Publication No. (SMA) 13-4760 DAWN Series D-39.

24. Qureshi AI, Suri MF, Guterman LR, et al. Cocaine use and the likelihood of nonfatal myocardial infarction and stroke: data from the Third National Health and Nutrition Examination Survey. Circulation 2001;103(4):502–6.

25. Caponnetto P, Auditore R, Russo C, et al. Dangerous relationships: asthma and substance abuse. J Addict Dis 2013;32(2):158–67.

26. Tseng W, Sutter ME, Albertson TE. Stimulants and the lung. Clin Rev Allergy Immunol 2014;46(1):82–100.

27. Boghdadi MS, Henning RJ. Cocaine: pathophysiology and clinical toxicology. Heart Lung 1997;26(6):466–83.

28. Fernandez WG, Hung O, Bruno GR, et al. Factors predictive of acute renal failure and need for hemodialysis among ED patients with rhabdomyolysis. Am J Emerg Med 2005;23(1):1–7.

29. Spronk DB, Van Wel JHP, Ramaekers JG, et al. Characterizing the cognitive effects of cocaine: a comprehensive review. Neurosci Biobehav Rev 2013;37: 1838–59.

30. Frazer KM, Richards Q, Keith DR. The long-term effects of cocaine use on cognitive functioning: a systematic critical review. Behav Brain Res 2018;348:241–62.

31. Blaho K, Logan B, Winbery S, et al. Blood cocaine and metabolite concentrations, clinical findings and outcome of patients presenting to an ED. Am J Emerg Med 2000;18:593–8.

32. Schwartz BG, Rezkalla S, Kloner RA. Cardiovascular effects of cocaine. Circulation 2010;122(24):2558–69.

33. Knight JR, Sherritt L, Schrier LA, et al. Validity of the CRAFFT substance abuse screening test among adolescent clinic patients. Arch Pediatr Adolesc Med 2002;156:607–14.

34. Levy S, Weiss R, Sherritt L, et al. An electronic screen for triaging adolescent substance use by risk levels. JAMA Pediatr 2014;168(9):822–8.

35. National Institute on Alcohol Abuse and Alcoholism (US). Alcohol screening and brief intervention for youth: a practitioner's guide. Bethesda (MD): National Institute on Alcohol Abuse and Alcoholism, US Department of Health and Human Services, National Institutes of Health; 2011.

36. Goldenring J, Cohen E. Getting into adolescent heads: an essential update. Contemp Pediatr 2004;21(1):1–19.

37. Kandel DB, Davies M, Karus D, et al. The consequences in young adulthood of adolescent drug involvement: an overview. Arch Gen Psychiatry 1986;43(8):746–54.

38. Levy SJ, Williams JF, Ryan SA, et al. Substance use, brief intervention, and referral to treatment. Pediatrics 2016;138:e20161211.

39. Dackis CA, O'Brien CP. Cocaine dependence: a disease of the brain's reward centers. J Subst Abuse Treat 2001;21(3):111–7.

40. Caywood K, Riggs P, Novins D. Adolescent substance use disorder prevention and treatment. Colorado Journal of Psychiatry and Psychology: Child and Adolescent Mental Health 2015;1(1):42–9.

41. Miller WR, Rollnick S. Motivational interviewing: preparing people to change addictive behavior. New York: Guilford Press; 1991.

42. Strickland JC, Stoops WW. The prevention and treatment of adolescent stimulant and methamphetamine use. Adolescent substance abuse. Cham (Switzerland): Springer; 2018. p. 233–60.

43. Waldron HB, Turner CW. Evidence-based psychosocial treatments for adolescent substance abuse. J Clin Child Adolesc Psychol 2008;37(1):238–61.

44. Carroll KM, Ball SA, Nich C, et al. Computer-assisted delivery of cognitive-behavioral therapy for addiction: a randomized trial of CBT4CBT. Am J Psychiatry 2008;165(7):881–8.

45. Riggs P. Encompass: an integrated treatment intervention for adolescents with co-occurring psychiatric and substance use disorders. Scientific Proceedings of the American Academy of Child and adolescent Psychiatry 61st Annual Meeting (AACAP). San Diego, October 20, 2014.

46. Stanger C, Lansing AH, Budney AJ. Advances in research on contingency management for adolescent substance use. Child Adolesc Psychiatr Clin N Am 2016;25(4):645–59.

47. Farronato NS, Dursteler-Macfarland KM, Wiesbeck GA, et al. A systematic review comparing cognitive-behavioral therapy and contingency management for cocaine dependence. J Addict Dis 2013;32(3):274–87.

48. Yu CH, Tsao P, Jesuthasan JR, et al. Incentivizing health care behaviors in emerging adults: a systematic review. Patient Preference Adherence 2016;10:371.

49. Lott DC, Jencius S. Effectiveness of very low-cost contingency management in a community adolescent treatment program. Drug Alcohol Depend 2009;102(1–3): 162–5.
50. Baldwin SA, Christian S, Berkeljon A, et al. The effects of family therapies for adolescent delinquency and substance abuse: a meta-analysis. J Marital Fam Ther 2012;38(1):281–304.
51. Santisteban DA, Mena MP, McCabe BE. Preliminary results for an adaptive family treatment for drug abuse in Hispanic youth. J Fam Psychol 2011;25(4):610.

Section 2: Special Topics

Effects of Fetal Substance Exposure on Offspring Substance Use

Neil C. Dodge, PhD*, Joseph L. Jacobson, PhD,
Sandra W. Jacobson, PhD

KEYWORDS

- Adolescent substance use disorders • Prenatal alcohol exposure
- Prenatal alcohol and drug exposure • Adolescent alcohol • Cocaine • Cigarettes
- Marijuana • Substance abuse risk

KEY POINTS

- Prenatal exposure to alcohol, cigarettes, and illicit drugs is associated with physical, cognitive, and behavioral problems in offspring.
- Prenatal exposure to alcohol, cigarettes, and illicit drugs of abuse is also related to increased risk of offspring substance use and abuse in adolescence and young adulthood.
- Effects of prenatal exposure on offspring substance use may occur independently of postnatal exposure through parental/familial use.
- Effects of prenatal exposures on offspring substance use may be mediated by behavior problems in childhood and adolescence.

INTRODUCTION

The National Institutes of Health have identified substance use disorders (SUDs) as a major public health problem and noted that the prevalence of these disorders, which typically emerge during adolescence or young adulthood, is increasing. By the time they graduate high school, 70% of adolescents have tried alcohol, 50% an illegal drug, and ~40% smoked cigarettes.[1] Illegal drug use, including marijuana, exceeds smoking, which has been declining in high schoolers over the last 2 decades, as public

Disclosure: The authors declare no financial conflicts of interest. This work was supported by funding from the National Institutes of Health/National Institute on Alcohol Abuse and Alcoholism (R01 AA06966 and R01 AA09524) and from the Lycaki-Young Fund from the State of Michigan.
Department of Psychiatry and Behavioral Neurosciences, Wayne State University School of Medicine, 3901 Chrysler Service Drive, Suite 1-B, Detroit, MI 48201, USA
* Corresponding author.
E-mail address: neildodge@wayne.edu

disapproval for smoking has increased. Many factors have been identified that seem to influence whether an adolescent experiments with drugs. Adolescents with impulse control problems, depression, anxiety, and attention-deficit/hyperactivity disorder (ADHD) are more likely to use drugs. Availability of drugs within the community; peer drug use; and household violence, physical or emotional abuse, mental illness, or drug use also increase the risk of SUDs.[2]

Early initiation of drug use also is an important predictor of SUDs. Most individuals with an SUD initiated substance use before age 18 years.[3] Although 15% who start drinking by age 14 years eventually develop an alcohol use disorder, only 2.1% of those who wait until they are 21 years old do so.[4] Thus, adolescence is a critical period for development of SUDs.

The effects of environmental factors, such as parental substance use/abuse, peer exposure, and socioeconomic factors, on adolescent substance use are well documented; however, the impact of more distal factors, such as prenatal substance exposure, are less well understood. Further complicating the relation between prenatal exposure and offspring use is the fact that prenatal exposure is highly correlated with many of the same environmental factors commonly associated with adolescent substance use, thus making it difficult to separate the influence of prenatal versus postnatal risks on offspring. In addition, the mechanism by which prenatal substance exposure influences offspring substance use is not well understood. Data from animal studies have shown that prenatal exposure can sensitize offspring to the effects of alcohol and drugs and increase their preference for alcohol and drugs.[5–7] Prenatal substance exposure is also associated with a wide range of offspring behavior problems, such as aggression and delinquency, factors that are commonly found to be associated with adolescent substance use.

This article reviews the existing literature on effects of prenatal exposure to alcohol, nicotine, and drugs on offspring alcohol and drug use.

EFFECTS OF PRENATAL ALCOHOL AND DRUG EXPOSURE ON OFFSPRING DEVELOPMENT

Fetal alcohol spectrum disorders (FASDs) is the umbrella term used to describe the range of adverse outcomes associated with prenatal alcohol exposure (PAE),[8] including fetal alcohol syndrome (FAS), the most severe form of FASD; partial FAS (PFAS); and alcohol-related neurodevelopmental disorder, in which individuals fail to meet criteria for FAS and PFAS but show mild to moderate neurobehavioral deficits. Although many children with FAS and PFAS are intellectually disabled and often have behavioral problems, some perform in the low average to average intelligence quotient range.[9–11] Many neurocognitive and behavioral deficits associated with PAE have been identified, including poorer verbal learning,[12,13] number processing,[14,15] attention, and executive function,[16] slower cognitive processing speed,[17,18] and impaired eyeblink conditioning.[19]

Children prenatally exposed to alcohol show parent-reported and teacher-reported behavioral problems,[20,21] and more internalizing and externalizing problems,[22,23] even at low levels of exposure. One or more drinks per day during the first trimester are associated with an increased rate of conduct disorder in adolescents.[24,25] Consistent with the neurocognitive and behavioral effects, there is evidence of structural brain abnormalities in the cerebellum, parietal lobes, corpus callosum, and caudate nucleus,[26,27] as well as compromised white matter integrity.[28–31] In addition, functional neuroimaging studies have provided evidence of prenatal alcohol-related neural dysfunction in verbal learning,[32] working memory,[33] and number processing.[34,35] However, little is known about effects of PAE on SUDs.

By contrast to PAE, for which extensive research has shown cognitive impairment even at low levels of exposure, prenatal drug exposure has been linked primarily to problems in arousal and behavior.[36,37] Cognitive and executive function deficits have been detected only in children exposed at high levels.[38–41] Offspring exposed prenatally to cigarette smoking are more likely to be irritable and have a difficult temperament during infancy and poor self-regulation during childhood,[42] as well as increased risk for ADHD[43] and difficulties in self-regulation, such as aggressive behavior,[44,45] antisocial behavior,[46] and conduct problems,[47,48] during adolescence. Prenatal marijuana exposure is related to deficits in attention and memory, increases in impulsivity, and delinquent behavior in adolescence.[49–51] Prenatal cocaine exposure affects attention, working memory, inhibitory control, and emotion regulation.[52,53] It also is related to fussy and difficult temperament during infancy,[54] internalizing problems and depressive symptoms through age 15 years,[55,56] and externalizing problems in childhood and aggressive behaviors in adolescence.[57]

PRENATAL ALCOHOL, SMOKING, AND DRUG EXPOSURE EFFECTS ON OFFSPRING SUBSTANCE USE

Table 1 summarizes findings from several major studies that were the only ones, to the authors' knowledge, to examine the impact of prenatal substance exposure on alcohol and drug use beginning in adolescence.

Alcohol

In one of the first studies of prenatal alcohol on offspring drinking behaviors, Baer and colleagues[58] reported that PAE predicted a composite measure of alcohol consumption and alcohol-related problems at age 14 years, whereas family history of alcohol problems did not. This effect persisted after control for family history, prenatal smoking, current parental drinking, and environmental potential confounders. At 21 years, PAE continued to predict offspring drinking problems, even after control for family history, other prenatal exposures, postnatal parental drinking, and other sociodemographic factors.[59] However, quantity and frequency of drinking at 21 years were not related to PAE.

Data from the Mater University Study of Pregnancy, a large prospectively recruited population-based birth cohort, showed that maternal consumption of more than 3 glasses of alcohol a few times per month in early pregnancy was related to a 3-fold increase in the risk for early-onset (13–17 years of age) and late-onset (18–21 years) alcohol use disorders.[60] Postnatal maternal alcohol consumption of 3 drinks or more was also associated with a 1.5-fold increase in the risk of late-onset alcohol use disorders. No significant effects were seen in offspring of mothers who consumed alcohol in late pregnancy. Offspring born to mothers who consumed 3 glasses of alcohol or more during pregnancy were 2.7 times more likely to have reported drinking 3 drinks or more at age 14 years, after controlling for prepregnancy and postpregnancy drinking.[61]

The Maternal Health Practices and Child Development (MHPCD) project is a large, prospectively recruited cohort based in Pittsburgh.[49] In the MHPCD cohort, detailed interviews of maternal alcohol, cigarette, and drug use were obtained from the pregnant mothers, and offspring were followed up multiple times through 22 years. Heavy first-trimester PAE had a direct effect on alcohol consumption in the offspring at 16 years, which was not mediated by childhood externalizing problems.[62] Similarly,

Table 1
Impact of prenatal substance exposure on alcohol and drug use beginning in adolescence

Author	Age (y)	Prenatal Exposure	Findings
Baer et al,[58] 1998	14	Alcohol	PAE more predictive of adolescent alcohol use and its negative consequences than family history of alcoholism. PAE effect remained significant after control for family history and other prenatal and environmental covariates
Cornelius et al,[66] 2000	16	Alcohol	First trimester alcohol exposure had direct effect on alcohol consumption in 16-y-old offspring
Cornelius et al,[66] 2000	10	Tobacco	Offspring exposed to >1 to 2 packs cigarettes/d had 5.5-fold increased risk for early tobacco use
Baer et al,[59] 2003	21	Alcohol	PAE related to alcohol use problems in young adults and persisted after control for other prenatal exposures and environmental covariates. PAE not related to amount of alcohol use after control for covariates
Porath & Fried,[70] 2005	16–21	Tobacco and marijuana	Offspring exposed to cigarettes >2 times as likely to initiate cigarette smoking. Prenatal marijuana–exposed offspring at increased risk for both tobacco and marijuana initiation
Cornelius et al,[67] 2005	14	Tobacco	Third trimester cigarette exposure associated with increased adolescent smoking; effect did not persist after control for current maternal smoking
Day et al,[71] 2006	14	Marijuana	Prenatal marijuana exposure predicted onset and frequency of marijuana use in 14-y-old offspring. Effects persisted after control for family history, current alcohol and tobacco use, pubertal stage, sexual activity, and home environment
Lundahl et al,[64] 2007	14	Alcohol	Prenatal and not postnatal alcohol exposure predicted adolescent use of alcohol and marijuana
Alati et al,[61] 2008	14	Alcohol	Offspring of mothers who consumed >3 glasses of alcohol prenatally at increased risk of reporting drinking >3 glasses of alcohol
Dodge et al,[65] 2009	19	Alcohol	Prenatal alcohol predicted alcohol consumption in 19-y-old offspring
Frank et al,[73] 2011	16	Cocaine	Heavier intrauterine cocaine exposure related to greater likelihood to initiate use of any illicit substance, including alcohol and marijuana
Delaney-Black et al,[75] 2011	14	Cocaine	Prenatal and postnatal cocaine predicted cocaine use at 14 y
Goldschmidt et al,[68] 2012	16	Alcohol, tobacco, marijuana	Prenatal cigarette exposure related to early initiation of alcohol, marijuana, and tobacco use after control for other prenatal exposures. Prenatal alcohol and marijuana not associated with initiation of use

(continued on next page)

Table 1
(*continued*)

Author	Age (y)	Prenatal Exposure	Findings
Cornelius et al,[69] 2012	22	Tobacco	Prenatal cigarette exposure associated with higher rates of smoking and self-reported nicotine dependence symptoms, independent of current maternal smoking
Rando et al,[89] 2013	14–17	Cocaine	Lower gray matter volume in superior frontal gyrus and precuneus in prenatal cocaine–exposed offspring. Lower gray matter volumes in these regions increased probability of substance use
Richardson et al,[55] 2013	15	Cocaine	First trimester cocaine exposure predicted earlier adolescent marijuana and alcohol initiation
Min et al,[76] 2014	15	Cocaine	Adolescents with prenatal cocaine exposure 2.8 times more likely to have SUDs
Minnes et al,[41] 2014	15	Cocaine	Prenatal cocaine–exposed adolescents twice as likely to use tobacco, 2.2 times more likely to use alcohol, and 1.8 times more likely to use marijuana
O'Brien & Hill,[90] 2015	13–22	Alcohol and tobacco	PAE associated with increased risk of cigarette use and SUDs. Prenatal cigarettes associated with increased adolescent cigarette use
Sonon et al,[72] 2015	22	Marijuana	Offspring exposed to marijuana more likely to be frequent marijuana users after control for prenatal alcohol, offspring race, sex, and age
Richardson et al,[74] 2019	21	Cocaine	Prenatal cocaine associated with early initiation of marijuana
Goldschmidt et al,[63] 2019	22	Alcohol	First trimester alcohol exposure associated with increased offspring alcohol use

at 22 years, first-trimester alcohol exposure was related to increased offspring alcohol use.[63] The Detroit Longitudinal Prenatal Alcohol Cohort[11] is another large, prospectively recruited cohort that assessed effects of PAE on offspring development. Data from the 14-year follow-up[64] showed that PAE and not postnatal maternal alcohol use was associated with increased alcohol and marijuana use among the 14-year-olds (**Table 2**). Adolescent alcohol use at 14 years subsequently predicted alcohol and drug use in these offspring at 19 years, indicating that the vulnerability of adolescent alcohol and drug use to PAE predicts greater use as the offspring reach young adulthood.[65]

Tobacco

In the MHPCD cohort, prenatal cigarette exposure increased the risk of early cigarette experimentation in 10-year-olds.[66] Offspring exposed to half a pack of cigarettes per day during pregnancy had a 5.5-fold increased risk for early tobacco experimentation. Effects of prenatal cigarette exposure on early experimentation had both a significant direct effect and an indirect effect through child behavior and peer tobacco use. At 14 years, third-trimester cigarette exposure was associated with adolescent smoking after control for other prenatal exposures, demographic variables, and maternal and child mental disorders.[67] However, after

Table 2
Relation of prenatal and postnatal alcohol exposure to adolescent substance use in the Detroit Longitudinal Prenatal Alcohol Cohort Study

	Prenatal						Postnatal	
	oz AA/d		oz AA/ Drinking Day		Frequency		oz AA/d	
	r	β	r	β	r	β	r	β
Alcohol (oz AA)								
Lifetime	0.08	0.06	0.14[b]	0.14[b]	0.07	0.06	−0.00	−0.01
Year	0.09	0.09	0.13[b]	0.14[b]	0.11[a]	0.13[a]	−0.02	−0.03
Month	0.09	0.09	0.02	0.03	0.13[b]	0.14[b]	−0.02	−0.04
Week	0.08	0.05	0.07	0.06	0.08	0.07	−0.18	−0.13[a]
Cigarettes								
Month	0.08	0.03	0.14[b]	0.12	0.07	0.04	−0.01	−0.03
Week	0.07	0.03	0.14[b]	0.12	0.07	0.04	−0.01	−0.03
Marijuana (occasions)								
Lifetime	0.05	0.00	0.12[a]	0.08	0.01	−0.03	−0.00	0.01
Year	0.01	−0.03	0.11[a]	0.08	−0.01	−0.03	−0.01	0.01
Month	0.08	0.05	0.15[b]	0.14[b]	0.07	0.07	−0.07	−0.07

Values are Pearson r and standardized regression coefficients (β), adjusted for confounding variables.
  1 standard drink is equivalent to 0.5 oz of absolute alcohol.
  Abbreviation: AA, absolute alcohol.
  [a] $P<.10$.
  [b] $P<.05$.

controlling for current maternal cigarette use and peer smoking, effects of prenatal cigarette exposure no longer predicted adolescent smoking at age 14 years. At age 16 years, adolescents exposed to tobacco during the first trimester were 1.4 times more likely to initiate use of multiple substances (cigarettes, alcohol, and/or marijuana) by age 16 years, whereas prenatal alcohol and marijuana exposure were not associated with early initiation of cigarettes, alcohol, and marijuana.[68] At 22 years, prenatal cigarette exposure was associated with higher rates of smoking and self-reported nicotine dependence symptoms, an effect that was independent of current maternal smoking.[69] Prenatal cigarette exposure was also associated with externalizing and internalizing problems and a history of criminal arrests. Prenatal alcohol and marijuana exposures were not associated with rates of smoking and self-reported nicotine dependence.[69]

The Ottawa Prenatal Prospective Study (OPPS) was a prospectively recruited longitudinal cohort designed to assess effects of maternal drug use in a low-risk, white, middle-class sample.[70] Adolescent cigarette and marijuana use was assessed in 152 individuals from 16 to 21 years old. Offspring born to mothers who smoked during pregnancy were more than twice as likely to have initiated cigarette use; however, prenatal smoking was not related to adolescent cigarettes smoked per day, initiation of marijuana use, or amount of daily use.

Marijuana

In the MHPCD project, prenatal marijuana exposure was associated with an earlier age of onset and frequency of marijuana use among 14-year-olds.[71] Those exposed to 1 joint per day of marijuana during gestation were 1.3 times more likely to have a higher frequency of marijuana use at age 14 years than those not exposed to marijuana, effects that persisted after control for current adolescent alcohol and tobacco use and peer drug use. Of note, the effect of prenatal marijuana exposure was specific to adolescent marijuana use and not related to adolescent smoking or alcohol use. At 22 years, offspring exposed to marijuana were more likely to be frequent marijuana users, after controlling for prenatal alcohol, offspring race, sex, and age,[72] whereas family history of substance use problems did not predict offspring marijuana use.

In the OPPS cohort, adolescents born to mothers who smoked marijuana during pregnancy were 2.5 times as likely to have initiated cigarette use and more than twice as likely to engage in daily cigarette use.[70] Those born to mothers who smoked marijuana were almost 3 times as likely to have initiated marijuana use, and joints per day of prenatal marijuana exposure were directly associated with the adolescent's report of joints per day.

Cocaine

Prenatal cocaine exposure has been found to be associated with earlier initiation of any substance, more than any other prenatal exposure. Intrauterine cocaine exposure was associated with earlier initiation of a licit or illicit substance at age 16 years.[73] These findings persisted after control for demographic background and other prenatal and postnatal exposures. Similarly, in the Pittsburgh longitudinal cohort, first-trimester cocaine exposure was related to earlier initiation of marijuana and alcohol in 15-year-olds.[55] By 21 years, prenatal cocaine exposure was a significant predictor of marijuana use initiation and amount of marijuana used in the past year[74]; it was also associated with higher odds of ever having been arrested and poorer inhibitory control. In a large Detroit longitudinal cohort, both prenatal and postnatal cocaine exposure were independently associated with adolescent cocaine use at age 14 years.[75] In a Cleveland cohort, 15-year-olds with prenatal cocaine exposure were more likely to have externalizing problems and were 2.8 times more likely to have substance use–related problems[76] and twice as likely to have used alcohol, cigarettes, or cocaine.[41]

SUMMARY

These studies show that prenatal exposure to alcohol and/or drugs can affect the risk of alcohol and drug use among exposed offspring. There is ample evidence that these more distal prenatal effects persist after controlling for other more proximal environmental factors, including current parental use and the home environment, suggesting that they are independent of the effects of the postnatal environment. Two possible mechanisms for how prenatal alcohol/drug exposure affect offspring use of alcohol and drugs are:

- Prenatal exposures may sensitize offspring to the rewarding effects of alcohol and drugs.
- Prenatal exposures increase the risk of offspring substance use, possibly through behavioral mediators such as childhood and adolescent behavior problems.

Data from animal models have shown a relation between gestational exposure to alcohol and drugs and increased preference for alcohol and drugs in offspring. Rodents prenatally exposed to alcohol consume more alcohol than unexposed controls,[5,77,78] and these results are consistent with those seen in humans. Among humans, young adults prenatally exposed to alcohol were more likely to rate alcohol as having a pleasant odor.[79] This enhanced alcohol preference, which is present in rat pups and persists into adolescence,[77,80] may be related to sensitization in the reward system because sucrose intake was also increased in the prenatally exposed rodents. Prenatal nicotine exposure is associated with increased nicotine self-administration[6] and increases the number of nicotine-binding sites in the brain.[81] Prenatal cocaine exposure has been shown to increase cocaine self-administration in rats,[7] and, in mice, increasing the dose of gestational cocaine increases the probability of acquiring cocaine self-administration.[82] Cocaine-exposed mice are also more sensitive to the locomotor effects of acute cocaine administration.[83] The increased preference and sensitization found in prenatally exposed rodents is likely driven by changes in the brain reward system. Morphologic and neurochemical changes to the midbrain areas mediating reward have been detected in prenatal alcohol, cigarette, and cocaine exposure.[84,85]

Prenatal exposure to alcohol and drugs is also associated with behavior problems that are associated with adolescent and young adult substance use. A consistent finding among prenatal alcohol, cocaine, and cigarette smoke exposure is increased externalizing behaviors and impulsivity in childhood and adolescence.[22,23,43,76,86–88] These behavioral problems in childhood and adolescence are also predictive of initiation of substance use and increased risk of substance-related problems. Thus, the relation between prenatal exposures and offspring substance use may also be mediated through behavior problems.

In summary, there is evidence that the fetal environment has an important impact on the development of SUDs in adolescence and adulthood. Longitudinal studies that extend well into adulthood are needed to determine the persistence, severity, and consequences of substance use problems in humans prenatally exposed to alcohol and/or drugs.

REFERENCES

1. Johnston LD, Miech RA, O'Malley PM, et al. Monitoring the Future national survey results on drug use, 1975-2017: overview, key findings on adolescent drug use. Ann Arbor (MI): Institute for Social Research, University of Michigan; 2018.

2. Sussman S, Skara S, Ames SL. Substance abuse among adolescents. Subst Use Misuse 2008;43:1802–28.

3. Dennis M, Babor TF, Roebuck C, et al. Changing the focus: the case for recognizing and treating cannabis use disorders. Addiction 2002;97:4–15.

4. Substance Abuse and Mental Health Services Administration (SAMHSA). Results from the 2012 national survey on drug use and health: summary of national findings. NSDUH series H-46, HHS publication No. (SMA) 13-4795. Rockville (MD): SAMHSA; 2013.

5. Spear NE, Molina JC. Fetal or infantile exposure to ethanol promotes ethanol ingestion in adolescence and adulthood: a theoretical review. Alcohol Clin Exp Res 2005;29:909–29.

6. Slotkin TA. If nicotine is a developmental neurotoxicant in animal studies, dare we recommend nicotine replacement therapy in pregnant women and adolescents? Neurotoxicol Teratol 2008;30:1–19.

7. Keller RW, Lefevre R, Raucci J, et al. Enhanced cocaine self-adminstration in adult rats prenatally exposed to cocaine. Neurosci Lett 1996;205:153–6.

8. Hoyme HE, May PA, Kalberg WO, et al. A practical clinical approach to diagnosis of fetal alcohol spectrum disorders: clarification of the 1996 institute of medicine criteria. Pediatrics 2005;115:39–47.

9. Streissguth AP, Aase JM, Clarren SK, et al. Fetal alcohol syndrome in adolescents and adults. JAMA 1991;265:1961–7.
10. Streissguth AP, Barr HM, Sampson PD. Moderate prenatal alcohol exposure: effects on child IQ and learning problems at age 7 1/2 years. Alcohol Clin Exp Res 1990;14:662–9.
11. Jacobson SW, Jacobson JL, Sokol RJ, et al. Maternal age, alcohol abuse history, and quality of parenting as moderators of the effects of prenatal alcohol exposure on 7.5-year intellectual function. Alcohol Clin Exp Res 2004;28:1732–45.
12. Lewis CE, Thomas KG, Dodge NC, et al. Verbal learning and memory impairment in children with fetal alcohol spectrum disorders. Alcohol Clin Exp Res 2015;39: 724–32.
13. Mattson SN, Riley EP, Delis DC, et al. Verbal learning and memory in children with fetal alcohol syndrome. Alcohol Clin Exp Res 1996;20:810–6.
14. Goldschmidt L, Richardson GA, Stoffer DS, et al. Prenatal alcohol exposure and academic achievement at age six: a nonlinear fit. Alcohol Clin Exp Res 1996;20: 763–70.
15. Jacobson JL, Dodge NC, Burden MJ, et al. Number processing in adolescents with prenatal alcohol exposure and ADHD: differences in the neurobehavioral phenotype. Alcohol Clin Exp Res 2011;35:431–42.
16. Coles CD, Platzman KA, Raskind-Hood CL, et al. A comparison of children affected by prenatal alcohol exposure and attention deficit, hyperactivity disorder. Alcohol Clin Exp Res 1997;21:150–61.
17. Jacobson SW, Jacobson JL, Sokol RJ, et al. Prenatal alcohol exposure and infant information processing ability. Child Dev 1993;64:1706–21.
18. Jacobson SW, Jacobson JL, Sokol RJ. Effects of fetal alcohol exposure on infant reaction time. Alcohol Clin Exp Res 1994;18:1125–32.
19. Jacobson SW, Stanton ME, Molteno CD, et al. Impaired eyeblink conditioning in children with fetal alcohol syndrome. Alcohol Clin Exp Res 2008;32:365–72.
20. Brown RT, Coles CD, Smith IE, et al. Effects of prenatal alcohol exposure at school age. II. Attention and behavior. Neurotoxicol Teratol 1991;13:369–76.
21. Carmichael Olson H, Streissguth AP, Sampson PD, et al. Association of prenatal alcohol exposure with behavioral and learning problems in early adolescence. J Am Acad Child Adolesc Psychiatry 1997;36:1187–94.
22. Dodge NC, Jacobson JL, Jacobson SW. Protective effects of the alcohol dehydrogenase-ADH1B*3 allele on attention and behavior problems in adolescents exposed to alcohol during pregnancy. Neurotoxicol Teratol 2014;41:43–50.
23. D'Onofrio BM, Van Hulle CA, Waldman ID, et al. Causal inferences regarding prenatal alcohol exposure and childhood externalizing problems. Arch Gen Psychiatry 2007;64:1296–304.
24. Disney ER, Iacono W, McGue M, et al. Strengthening the case: prenatal alcohol exposure is associated with increased risk for conduct disorder. Pediatrics 2008; 122:e1225–30.
25. Larkby CA, Goldschmidt L, Hanusa BH, et al. Prenatal alcohol exposure is associated with conduct disorder in adolescence: findings from a birth cohort. J Am Acad Child Adolesc Psychiatry 2011;50:262–71.
26. Archibald SL, Fennema-Notestine C, Gamst A, et al. Brain dysmorphology in individuals with severe prenatal alcohol exposure. Dev Med Child Neurol 2001;43: 148–54.
27. Lebel C, Roussotte F, Sowell ER. Imaging the impact of prenatal alcohol exposure on the structure of the developing human brain. Neuropsychol Rev 2011;21: 102–18.

28. Li L, Coles CD, Lynch ME, et al. Voxelwise and skeleton-based region of interest analysis of fetal alcohol syndrome and fetal alcohol spectrum disorders in young adults. Hum Brain Mapp 2009;30:3265–74.

29. Sowell ER, Johnson A, Kan E, et al. Mapping white matter integrity and neurobehavioral correlates in children with fetal alcohol spectrum disorders. J Neurosci 2008;28:1313–9.

30. Fan J, Jacobson SW, Taylor PA, et al. White matter deficits mediate effects of prenatal alcohol exposure on cognitive development in childhood. Hum Brain Mapp 2016;37:2943–58.

31. Treit S, Lebel C, Baugh L, et al. Longitudinal MRI reveals altered trajectory of brain development during childhood and adolescence in fetal alcohol spectrum disorders. J Neurosci 2013;33:10098–109.

32. O'Hare ED, Lu LH, Houston SM, et al. Altered frontal-parietal functioning during verbal working memory in children and adolescents with heavy prenatal alcohol exposure. Hum Brain Mapp 2009;30:3200–8.

33. Diwadkar VA, Meintjes EM, Goradia D, et al. Differences in cortico-striatal-cerebellar activation during working memory in syndromal and nonsyndromal children with prenatal alcohol exposure. Hum Brain Mapp 2013;34:1931–45.

34. Woods K, Meintjes EM, Molteno CD, et al. Parietal dysfunction during number processing in children with fetal alcohol spectrum disorders. Neuroimage Clin 2015;8:594–605.

35. Santhanam P, Li Z, Hu X, et al. Effects of prenatal alcohol exposure on brain activation during an arithmetic task: an fMRI study. Alcohol Clin Exp Res 2009;33:1901–8.

36. Tronick EZ, Frank DA, Cabral H, et al. Late dose-response effects of prenatal cocaine exposure on newborn neurobehavioral performance. Pediatrics 1996;98:76.

37. Singer LT, Minnes S, Min MO, et al. Prenatal cocaine exposure and child outcomes: a conference report based on a prospective study from Cleveland. Hum Psychopharmacol 2015;30:285–9.

38. Jacobson SW, Jacobson JL, Sokol RJ, et al. New evidence for neurobehavioral effects of in utero cocaine exposure. J Pediatr 1996;129:581–90.

39. Singer LT, Arendt R, Minnes S, et al. Developing language skills of cocaine-exposed infants. Pediatrics 2001;107:1057–64.

40. Frank DA, McCarten KM, Robson CD, et al. Level of in utero cocaine exposure and neonatal ultrasound findings. Pediatrics 1999;104:1101.

41. Minnes S, Singer L, Min MO, et al. Effects of prenatal cocaine/polydrug exposure on substance use by age 15. Drug Alcohol Depend 2014;134:201–10.

42. Stroud LR, Paster RL, Goodwin MS, et al. Maternal smoking during pregnancy and neonatal behavior: a large-scale community study. Pediatrics 2009;123:e842–8.

43. Button TMM, Thapar A, McGuffin P. Relationship between antisocial behaviour, attention-deficit hyperactivity disorder and maternal prenatal smoking. Br J Psychiatry 2005;187:155–60.

44. Brion MJ, Victora C, Matijasevich A, et al. Maternal smoking and child psychological problems: disentangling causal and noncausal effects. Pediatrics 2010;126:e57–65.

45. Day NL, Richardson GA, Goldschmidt L, et al. Effects of prenatal tobacco exposure on preschoolers' behavior. J Dev Behav Pediatr 2000;21:180–8.

46. Wakschlag LS, Hans SL. Maternal smoking during pregnancy and conduct problems in high-risk youth: a developmental framework. Dev Psychopathol 2002;14:351–69.

47. Baler RD, Volkow ND, Fowler JS, et al. Is fetal brain monoamine oxidase inhibition the missing link between maternal smoking and conduct disorders? J Psychiatry Neurosci 2008;33:187.

48. Wakschlag LS, Pickett KE, Kasza KE, et al. Is prenatal smoking associated with a developmental pattern of conduct problems in young boys? J Am Acad Child Adolesc Psychiatry 2006;45:461–7.

49. Day NL, Richardson GA, Goldschmidt L, et al. Effect of prenatal marijuana exposure on the cognitive development of offspring at age three. Neurotoxicol Teratol 1994;16:169–75.

50. Fried PA, Watkinson B, Gray R. A follow-up study of attentional behavior in 6-year-old children exposed prenatally to marihuana, cigarettes, and alcohol. Neurotoxicol Teratol 1992;14:299–311.

51. Goldschmidt L, Richardson GA, Cornelius MD, et al. Prenatal marijuana and alcohol exposure and academic achievement at age 10. Neurotoxicol Teratol 2004;26:521–32.

52. Carmody DP, Bennett DS, Lewis M. The effects of prenatal cocaine exposure and gender on inhibitory control and attention. Neurotoxicol Teratol 2011;33:61–8.

53. Mayes L, Snyder PJ, Langlois E, et al. Visuospatial working memory in school-aged children exposed in utero to cocaine. Child Neuropsychol 2007;13:205–18.

54. Richardson GA, Goldschmidt L, Willford J. The effects of prenatal cocaine use on infant development. Neurotoxicol Teratol 2008;30:96–106.

55. Richardson GA, Larkby C, Goldschmidt L, et al. Adolescent initiation of drug use: effects of prenatal cocaine exposure. J Am Acad Child Adolesc Psychiatry 2013;52:37–46.

56. Richardson GA, Goldschmidt L, Larkby C, et al. Effects of prenatal cocaine exposure on adolescent development. Neurotoxicol Teratol 2015;49:41–8.

57. Richardson GA, Goldschmidt L, Leech S, et al. Prenatal cocaine exposure: effects on mother-and teacher-rated behavior problems and growth in school-age children. Neurotoxicol Teratol 2011;33:69–77.

58. Baer JS, Barr HM, Bookstein FL, et al. Prenatal alcohol exposure and family history of alcoholism in the etiology of adolescent alcohol problems. J Stud Alcohol 1998;59:533–43.

59. Baer JS, Sampson PD, Barr HM, et al. A 21-year longitudinal analysis of the effects of prenatal alcohol exposure on young adult drinking. Arch Gen Psychiatry 2003;60:377–85.

60. Alati R, Al Mamun A, Williams GM, et al. In utero alcohol exposure and prediction of alcohol disorders in early adulthood: a birth cohort study. Arch Gen Psychiatry 2006;63:1009–16.

61. Alati R, Clavarino A, Najman JM, et al. The developmental origin of adolescent alcohol use: findings from the Mater University Study of Pregnancy and its outcomes. Drug Alcohol Depend 2008;98:136–43.

62. Cornelius MD, De Genna NM, Goldschmidt L, et al. Prenatal alcohol and other early childhood adverse exposures: direct and indirect pathways to adolescent drinking. Neurotoxicol Teratol 2016;55:8–15.

63. Goldschmidt L, Richardson GA, De Genna NM, et al. Prenatal alcohol exposure and offspring alcohol use and misuse at 22 years of age: a prospective longitudinal study. Neurotoxicol Teratol 2019;71:1–5.

64. Lundahl LH, Jacobson SW, Dodge NC, et al. Relation of early adolescent alcohol use to prenatal alcohol exposure. Alcohol Clin Exp Res 2007;31:185A.

65. Dodge NC, Lundahl LH, Morrison AL, et al. Prenatal alcohol exposure predicts greater alcohol use in young adulthood, after control for confounding variables. Alcohol Clin Exp Res 2009;33:39A.

66. Cornelius MD, Leech SL, Goldschmidt L, et al. Prenatal tobacco exposure: is it a risk factor for early tobacco experimentation? Nicotine Tob Res 2000;2:45–52.

67. Cornelius MD, Leech SL, Goldschmidt L, et al. Is prenatal tobacco exposure a risk factor for early adolescent smoking? A follow-up study. Neurotoxicol Teratol 2005;27:667–76.

68. Goldschmidt L, Cornelius MD, Day NL. Prenatal cigarette smoke exposure and early initiation of multiple substance use. Nicotine Tob Res 2012;14:694–702.

69. Cornelius MD, Goldschmidt L, De Genna NM, et al. Long-term effects of prenatal cigarette smoke exposure on behavior dysregulation among 14-year-old offspring of teenage mothers. Matern Child Health J 2012;16:694–705.

70. Porath AJ, Fried PA. Effects of prenatal cigarette and marijuana exposure on drug use among offspring. Neurotoxicol Teratol 2005;27:267–77.

71. Day NL, Goldschmidt L, Thomas CA, et al. Prenatal marijuana exposure contributes to the prediction of marijuana use at age 14. Addiction 2006;101:1313–22.

72. Sonon KE, Richardson GA, Cornelius JR, et al. Prenatal marijuana exposure predicts marijuana use in young adulthood. Neurotoxicol Teratol 2015;47:10–5.

73. Frank DA, Rose-Jacobs KA, Crooks D, et al. Adolescent initiation of licit and illicit substance use: impact of intrauterine exposures and post-natal exposure to violence. Neurotoxicol Teratol 2011;33:100–9.

74. Richardson GA, De Genna NM, Goldschmidt L, et al. Prenatal cocaine exposure: direct and indirect associations with 21-year-old offspring substance use and behavior problems. Drug Alcohol Depend 2019;195:121–31.

75. Delaney-Black V, Chiodo LM, Hannigan JH, et al. Prenatal and postnatal cocaine exposure predict teen cocaine use. Neurotoxicol Teratol 2011;33:110–9.

76. Min MO, Minnes S, Lang A, et al. Externalizing behavior and substance use related problems at 15 years in prenatally cocaine exposed adolescents. J Adolesc 2014;37:269–79.

77. Chotro MG, Arias C. Prenatal exposure to ethanol increases ethanol consumption: a conditioned response? Alcohol 2003;30:19–28.

78. Arias C, Chotro MG. Increased preference for ethanol in the infant rat after prenatal ethanol exposure, expressed on intake and taste reactivity tests. Alcohol Clin Exp Res 2005;29:337–46.

79. Hannigan JH, Chiodo LM, Sokol RJ, et al. Prenatal alcohol exposure selectively enhances young adult perceived pleasantness of alcohol odors. Physiol Behav 2015;148:71–7.

80. Domínguez HD, López MF, Molina JC. Neonatal responsiveness to alcohol odor and infant alcohol intake as a function of alcohol experience during late gestation. Alcohol 1998;16:109–17.

81. Hellström-Lindahl E, Nordberg A. Smoking during pregnancy: a way to transfer the addiction to the next generation? Respiration 2002;69:289–93.

82. Rocha BA, Mead AN, Kosofsky BE. Increased vulnerability to self-administer cocaine in mice prenatally exposed to cocaine. Psychopharmacology (Berl) 2002;163:221–9.

83. Crozatier C, Guerriero RM, Mathieu F, et al. Altered cocaine-induced behavioral sensitization in adult mice exposed to cocaine in utero. Brain Res Dev Brain Res 2003;147:97–105.

84. Lidow MS. Consequences of prenatal cocaine exposure in nonhuman primates. Brain Res Dev Brain Res 2003;147:23–36.
85. Malanga CJ, Kosofsky BE. Does drug abuse beget drug abuse? Behavioral analysis of addiction liability in animal models of prenatal drug exposure. Brain Res Dev Brain Res 2003;147:47–57.
86. Bada HS, Das A, Bauer CR, et al. Impact of prenatal cocaine exposure on child behavior problems through school age. Pediatrics 2007;119:e348–59.
87. Bendersky M, Lewis M. Prenatal cocaine exposure and impulse control at two years. Ann N Y Acad Sci 1998;846:365–7.
88. Ernst M, Moolchan ET, Robinson ML. Behavioral and neural consequences of prenatal exposure to nicotine. J Am Acad Child Adolesc Psychiatry 2001;40:630–41.
89. Rando K, Chaplin TM, Potenza MN, et al. Prenatal cocaine exposure and gray matter volume in adolescent boys and girls: relationship to substance use initiation. Biol Psychiatr 2013;74:482–9.
90. O'Brien JW, Hill SY. Effects of prenatal alcohol and cigarette exposure on offspring substance use in multiplex, alcohol-dependent families. Alcohol Clin Exp Res 2015;38:2952–61.

Behavioral Addictions

Excessive Gambling, Gaming, Internet, and Smartphone Use Among Children and Adolescents

Jeffrey L. Derevensky, PhD*, Victoria Hayman, BSc,
Lynette Gilbeau, BEd

KEYWORDS

- Behavioral disorders • Gambling • Gaming • Internet addiction • Smartphone use

KEY POINTS

- The introduction of behavioral addictions is a relatively new concept in psychiatry. Although many of the disorders subsumed under the term behavioral addictions have existed for decades, it was not until 2010 that the DSM workgroup, based on a growing body of literature, suggested adding the term *behavioral addictions* to their official classification of psychiatric diagnoses in the *Diagnostic and Statistical Manual of Mental Disorders, Fifth Edition*.
- Gambling, typically thought to be an adult behavior, has become commonplace among adolescents.
- Although technological advances have made accessing information and communication easier, excessive use of the Internet and smartphones can result in multiple mental and physical health issues.
- Gambling disorders, gaming disorders, Internet use disorder, and excessive smartphone use often begin during childhood and adolescence.

BEHAVIORAL ADDICTIONS

The introduction of behavioral addictions is a relatively new concept in psychiatry.[1] Although many of the disorders subsumed under the term behavioral addictions have existed for decades, it was not until 2010 that the DSM workgroup, based on a growing body of literature, suggested adding the term *behavioral addictions* to their official classification of psychiatric diagnoses in the *Diagnostic and Statistical Manual of Mental Disorders, Fifth Edition* (DSM-5).[2] There was strong empirical support

---

International Centre for Youth Gambling Problems and High-Risk Behaviors, McGill University, 3724 McTavish Street, Montreal, Quebec H3A 1Y2, Canada
* Corresponding author.
E-mail address: Jeffrey.derevensky@mcgill.ca

Pediatr Clin N Am 66 (2019) 1163–1182
https://doi.org/10.1016/j.pcl.2019.08.008
0031-3955/19/© 2019 Elsevier Inc. All rights reserved.

indicating that a number of potentially risky behaviors, besides psychoactive substance ingestion, produce short-term rewards that may result in persistent behaviors despite the individual's understanding and awareness of adverse consequences.[3–6] The American Psychiatric Association (DSM-5),[2] World Health Organization (*International Classification of Diseases, Eleventh Revision* [ICD-11])[7] and the American Society of Addiction Medicine[8] have all recognized that such disorders, characterized as *behavioral addictions*, to varying degrees and with different, but similar, clinical criteria should be recognized.

Our current conceptualization of behavioral addictions is that those disorders under the rubric of behavioral addictions share many similarities and commonalities with other forms of addictive behaviors.[3] The DSM workgroup concluded that the emerging neuroscientific data supported a unified neurobiological theory of addictions independent of the specific substances, substrates, or activities, which should allow for the inclusion of behavioral addictions as well as chemical addictions.[1] Although a number of behavioral addictions were suggested for inclusion, the workgroup concluded that there was sufficient evidence for inclusion of a gambling disorder and that further research was necessary before including a gaming disorder, Internet use disorder, smartphone disorder, sex addiction, exercise addiction, and shopping addiction. The World Health Organization has nevertheless elected to include gaming disorder in its ICD-11.[7]

Behavioral addictions may be best understood from a biopsychosocial model.[1,9] The essential feature of behavioral addictions lies in the individual's failure to resist impulses, drives, or temptations, which if engaged in excessively may result in harmful consequences. Griffiths,[9] early on, articulated 6 core elements found among individuals experiencing a behavioral addiction; these being salience (the activity becomes highly valued and takes precedence over other activities), mood modification (the emotional response to the behavior; this may be in the form of an adrenalin rush when engaged in the behavior or may lead to a reduction in a depressive state), tolerance (the need for increasing amounts of the behavior to achieve the desired level of mood modification), withdrawal symptoms (unpleasant feelings or physiologic withdrawal symptoms when cutting down or stopping the activity), conflict (conflicts with other activities or persons due to the behavior), and relapse (a relatively high rate of returning back to the initial behavior). Each of these core elements can be found among all behavioral addictions.[10]

Although several behavioral addictions (eg, compulsive shopping, sexual addiction, smartphone addiction) seem to be more typical of middle age or even older adults, the onset of many of these behavioral disorders has been shown to occur during childhood, adolescence, and/or early adulthood. It may well be that the consequences and problems associated with a behavioral addiction may be more severe during adulthood, but the resulting problems associated with a behavioral addiction for children and adolescents also can be pervasive.

CHILD AND ADOLESCENT RISKY BEHAVIORS

Over the past few decades, there has been a significant and remarkable invigoration of both theoretic and empirical research on child and adolescent risk behaviors (those behaviors that if engaged in excessively can, directly or indirectly, compromise the individual's physical and mental health, and the life course trajectories of young people).[10–12] Today's conceptualizations of child and adolescent risky behaviors encompass a wide array of causal domains, including cultural, genetic, biological, social, psychological, and environmental factors.[11] Much of the early work focused on adolescent problematic behaviors (substance and alcohol abuse, cigarette smoking, unprotected sexual activity, drinking and driving, and delinquency), all of which had potentially serious negative short-term and long-term consequences for the individual, the individual's family, and society. These risky behaviors often compromise one's "healthy development," and result in mental health, social, educational, and in some cases legal difficulties for adolescents.[13] Given the pervasiveness of the problems, researchers and clinicians have sought a better understanding as to the reasons why individuals engage in these behaviors, their risk factors, both proximal and distal, as well as the identification and assessment of protective factors.[11] This has further led to issues related to prevention programs focused on harm minimization or harm reduction.[14]

As previously noted, although there is much commonality among different behavioral addictions, there also remains increasing evidence that different problem behaviors are associated with distinct risk factors, which is reflected in differential diagnoses applicable to specific mental health disorders occurring during childhood or adolescence.[2,7] Derevensky[10] argued that although it is important to study individuals displaying a single form of problem behavior, understanding youth displaying problems in multiple domains can significantly add to our knowledge. He points to Jacobs'[15] *General Theory of Addictions* suggesting that an addiction is a dependent state acquired over time to relieve stress. Jacobs[15] postulated that 2 interrelated sets of factors predispose individuals to addictions: (1) an abnormal physiologic resting state, and (2) childhood experiences producing a deep sense of inadequacy. The unipolar physiologic resting state (over or under stimulation) is a key factor within this theoretic model, suggesting that an addiction may be in part inherited through a genetic disposition. In an attempt to reduce or minimize the effects of this physiologic state, individuals, through maladaptive coping strategies, turn to some addictive behavior as a form of stress reduction.[15]

Although a large number of behavioral addictions have been clinically reported, this review focuses on gambling disorders (recognized in the DSM-5),[2] gaming disorders (recognized in ICD-11),[7] as well Internet addiction and excessive smartphone use, given these disorders appear to have emerged as important clinical and social issues.

GAMBLING DISORDERS

Society has witnessed a dramatic expansion of all forms of gambling. Once thought to be an activity only for adults, gambling has become a popular mainstream activity in most parts of the world along with its concomitant associated problems.[10,12] Whether purchasing lottery scratch cards with familiar themes, playing poker or other card games among friends, or wagering on sports, international studies have consistently reported that gambling has become part of the life experiences for large numbers of adolescents.[12,16–21]

Despite prohibitions from engaging in government-regulated gambling activities (the age varies based on the type of gambling and jurisdiction), adolescents have been reported to have engaged in all forms of gambling, including online gambling.[12,16,17,21,22] There is abundant evidence suggesting that a pattern of gambling behavior often occurs early, with children as young as ages 9 and 10 engaging in some form of gambling,[12,16–18,22,23] yet few parents,[24] teachers,[25,26] and even mental health professionals[27,28] perceive gambling to be a serious issue for youth. Although most youth who gamble can be best described as social, recreational, occasional, or infrequent gamblers, a small but identifiable number of adolescents develop a serious gambling problem.

With almost 80% of adolescents reporting having gambled for money at least once during their lifetime,[12] there is a growing concern that problem and disordered gambling among adolescents is a significant issue. Calado and colleagues,[16] in reviewing the adolescent gambling literature, reported that between 0.2% and 12.3% of youth meet criteria for problem gambling, notwithstanding assessment differences, cutoff scores, timeframes, accessibility, and availability of different gambling activities. They also suggested that in addition to male individuals being more likely to report gambling and experiencing problems, individuals who belong to an ethnic minority may be at a higher risk for problem/disordered gambling. Their analyses further revealed that youth engaged in online Internet wagering are more prone to experience gambling and gambling-related problems, likely the result of its easy accessibility, affordability, convenience, and anonymity.[16,19,29,30] It is important to note that youth with gambling problems typically do not elect to seek treatment for gambling problems.[10,12]

The types of gambling activities in which youth are engaged is often related to the accessibility and availability of specific forms of gambling. School age children are much more prone to engage in gambling activities among peers (often related to skill-related games), lottery tickets (eg, scratch-instant win tickets) and sports gambling. As they get older and have greater access to money and credit cards, they may begin to get involved in video lottery terminals (where available), casinos, and online gambling.[12]

Risk Factors Associated with a Gambling Disorder

There is a growing list of risk and protective factors associated with youth experiencing gambling problems. The cumulative body of gambling research suggests male individuals are more likely to engage in gambling and experience gambling problems,[12,16,31] they begin gambling at an earlier age,[32] they may be members of an ethnic minority,[33,34] may have had disrupted familial and peer relationships,[35] and have a parent or close family member with a gambling disorder.[12,32] From a psychological perspective, many of these adolescents, like their adult counterparts, report significant mental health issues, including anxiety disorders,[36] depression,[37–39] and impulsivity.[37] These individuals score lower on measures of conformity and self-discipline, and they report high rates of suicide ideation and attempts.[39,40] Academically, adolescents with gambling problems experience a wide variety of school-related problems, including impaired academic performance, interpersonal difficulties, and conduct-related problems.[12,41] Other factors associated with youth gambling problems include having a "big win" (this being dependent on their socioeconomic level and age of the individual),[32] with peer influences being predictive of gambling problems.[42]

Adolescent problem gamblers, like their adult counterparts, exhibit erroneous beliefs, their cognitive thinking lacks a knowledge of the independence of events, and they report an exaggerated level of skill when gambling. As well, they typically have poor or maladaptive general coping skills,[40,43] have a high-risk propensity,[14] and have poor resiliency in light of adversity.[44,45] In addition, adolescent problem gamblers report more daily hassles and traumatic life events.[46]

Despite these well-established risk factors and their associations with youth gambling problems, many children and adolescents never develop significant problems, suggesting that there are protective factors that play an important role in minimizing and decreasing the likelihood of youth problem gambling.[45] Several early studies by Dickson and her colleagues[14] revealed that low-risk propensity, family cohesion, school connectedness, achievement motivation, and effective coping skills served as protective factors. Lussier and colleagues[45] further reported on the importance of resilience being an important protective factor. Those youth having high scores on resiliency measures were significantly less likely to experience gambling problems. These factors may serve to counteract risk factors through a cancellation process.[14,44,45]

Assessing Gambling Problems Among Adolescents and Young Adults

Due to the growing awareness of gambling problems among adolescents, a number of instruments have been adapted from adult scales for this age group. The South Oaks Gambling Screen-Revised for Adolescents,[47] DSM-IV-J[48] and its revision the DSM-IV-MR-J,[49] and the Massachusetts Gambling Screen[50] have been used in a large number of adolescent prevalence studies. Each of these instruments was modeled on adult screening instruments; however, more recently, the Canadian Adolescent Gambling Inventory[51] was specifically developed to assess gambling severity among adolescents.

Like adult scales, common constructs underlie all the instruments. The notion of deception (lying), stealing money to support gambling, preoccupation, and chasing losses are common to all of these instruments. Similarly, although the number of items and constructs differ, each criterion item has equal weighting, and a cut score is provided identifying pathologic gambling for each respective instrument (see Derevensky[12] for a more comprehensive discussion and description of these instruments).

The Changing Face of Gambling

Gambling has dramatically changed during the past decade. Not only has it become more socially acceptable, easily accessible, and readily available, but technological innovations have revolutionized the industry and the way we gamble. Online gambling, wagering through one's smartphone, fantasy sports wagering, in-play and micro sports betting, are just a few examples. In some jurisdictions, Video Lottery Terminals are available on almost every corner, and sports wagering is prevalent. There is little doubt that youth, in spite of prohibitions, have managed to access and engage in many of these forms of gambling.[12] Recently, Derevensky and Gainsbury[52] raised concerns about social casino gaming; simulated forms of gambling that individuals play for points or chips but that may have higher than average payout rates. In a series of studies by Kim and colleagues,[53–55] there seems to be a crossover and migration from gambling on online social casino games to actual online gambling among young adults. King,[56] in reviewing the available literature, pointed to the convergence between gaming and gambling and suggested some forms of gaming may be a "gateway" to actual gambling. He concluded, after a review of the available empirical evidence, that simulated gambling during adolescence increases risk of monetary gambling during adulthood. McBride and Derevensky[57] also reported that social casino game playing among adolescents was related to more problematic gambling behaviors. Other forms of gambling, such as fantasy sports wagering, appear to be popular among adolescent boys. Those individuals engaging in these behaviors frequently were reported to experience a number of gambling-related behaviors.[58]

GAMING DISORDERS

With the appearance of electronic games in the 1990s and technological advances associated with game consoles and smartphones, video games and online gaming continue to increase in popularity and accessibility. There is evidence that more than 90% of children and adolescents in the United States play video games, with a large percentage spending an increasingly substantial amount of time playing.[59,60] Király and colleagues[61] argued that online video games are currently one of the most widespread recreational activities irrespective of culture, age, and gender. Newzoo[62] suggested that in spite of some concerns, the gaming market continues to grow and is expected to become a $180 billion market by 2021 (more than doubling in size since 2014). It should not be interpreted that gaming in and of itself is harmful. On the contrary, video games may satisfy certain psychological needs of the users, including identity expression, a sense of mastery and achievement, and the desire to escape from reality.[63] Despite some positive attributions associated with gaming, if done excessively, individuals can experience a number of negative consequences (eg, financial losses, as online games often require money to continue play, psychological detachment, sleep deprivation, eating and nutritional problems, a lack of personal and social interaction, depression, and anxiety, among others). Given its attractiveness, widespread popularity, easy accessibility and availability, it is not surprising that an identifiable number of individuals appear to engage in this behavior excessively. Although the DSM-5[2] Work Group identified gaming disorder as a potential disorder worthy of further investigation, the World Health Organization decided there was sufficient clinical and experimental evidence to include it in the ICD-11[7] as a behavioral disorder requiring treatment for individuals meeting the clinical criteria. A gaming disorder is defined as a pattern of gaming behavior ("digital gaming" or "video gaming") characterized by impaired control over gaming, and increased priority given to gaming over other activities, interests, and daily activities. It is marked by a continuation or escalation of gaming despite the occurrence of negative consequences. As part of the clinical criteria, this behavior is not episodic and must be of sufficient severity (both intensity and frequency) to result in significant impairment in personal, familial, social, educational, occupational, or other important areas of functioning. The World Health Organization diagnostic criteria also indicate that this behavior must be present for at least 12 months; however, in exceptional cases of a severe gaming disorder, a shorter timeframe is used.[7]

A consensus concerning prevalence rates of a gaming disorder has been difficult to achieve given significant variability among studies in terms of definition, assessment criteria, geographic considerations, accessibility (related to income and Internet access), and different methodological approaches. Several reviews of the literature examining the prevalence rates of gaming disorders[61,64,65] suggest that approximately 1.5% to 9.9% of adolescents appear to have a gaming disorder, with some research reporting rates as high as 25% among US university students.[66] Although adults can also exhibit symptoms of a gaming disorder, Kuss and Griffiths[67–69] concluded that gaming disorders are more typical among children and adolescents (possibly because of more free time). A recent study revealed that excessive gaming time may not only be gender-dependent but also dependent on the individual's preference of game genre.[70] Role-playing games and shooter-type games may be related to higher time spent gaming.[70] Eichenbaum and colleagues[71] reported that Massively Multiplayers Online Role-Playing Games were highly related to Internet gaming disorders, whereas action and puzzle games were found to be minimally linked to a gaming disorder.[72] However, if done excessively, these games can lead to a gaming disorder. One's motivation for gaming has also been shown to be related to a gaming disorder. For example, if gaming is primarily used for social reasons versus psychological escape, it may be less problematic. Nevertheless, as gaming frequency and play time escalate, the likelihood of a gaming disorder increases. In addition, the more game genres engaged in, the greater the incidence of a gaming disorder.[73]

Although there are several studies that have found an association between Internet use and a gaming disorder, those with a severe gaming disorder have a variety of psychosocial problems and psychiatric conditions (eg, depressive symptomatology, attention-deficit hyperactivity, mood disorders, anxiety disorders, personality disorders, and obsessive-compulsive disorders).[61,74–78] However, it is important to note that there is very little research examining the temporal or causal relationships between psychiatric disorders and gaming disorders.[79–82] Further, disordered gaming significantly predicted poorer academic performance, even after controlling for sex, age, and weekly amounts of game playing.[59] Long-term effects of violent games also seem to be predictive of more aggressive behavior.[83] Kuss and colleagues[84] further suggested that understanding one's cultural context is important, as it embeds gamers into a community with shared beliefs and practices, endowing their gaming with a particular meaning.

Whether it is due to gaming's social features, the ability to manipulate and control aspects of the game itself, reward and punishment features (eg, earning or losing points), the aesthetic quality of the games, the ability to assume an alternate identity with the game characters, or the ability to interact with others, children and adolescents are particularly drawn to these games.[67–69,85] Online gaming has become a space of "virtual socialization" in which players experience social interactions as an integral part of the gaming process.[78] For some, the increased frequency of gaming represents a need for completion of more intricate, time-consuming, or difficult goals to achieve satisfaction and the need to rectify perceived gaming inadequacies.[81]

Gaming: Some Recent Developments

One evolution of the gaming movement has been what is referred to as e-Sports, whereby individuals watch teams of gamers compete against each other in real time. These competitions have attracted tens of thousands of spectators, and some players have developed a strong cultlike following. This has resulted in an increase in young people reporting a desire to become "professional gamers." Collegiate and professional e-Sports (competitive video gaming) have become more organized and popular.[86,87] Since their establishment in the early 2000s, professional and club e-Sports have seen a rapid growth in both participation and viewership,[88,89] with some colleges and universities now offering scholarships for top players.[87] The gambling industry has now capitalized on this emerging market, with some casinos now accepting wagers on the outcome of the matches.

Assessing Internet Gaming Disorders

The need for common diagnostic criteria has been repeatedly emphasized in the psychological literature.[90] The existence of multiple instruments reflects the divergence of opinions in the field regarding how best to diagnose this condition. This has not precluded researchers from developing several scales, some of which include the Internet Gaming Disorder Test-20[91] and its short form (IGDS-9)[92] (assesses severity of online and offline gaming behaviors), Internet Gaming Disorder Test-10[61] (a 10-item scale based on the DMS-5 criteria for a gambling disorder), and the Internet Gaming Disorders Scales (both 9-item and 27-item versions).[93,94] All of these scales are designed to assess negative consequences associated with a gaming disorder.

INTERNET ADDICTION DISORDER

Similar to a gaming disorder, the American Psychiatric Association[2] suggested that Internet use disorder as an addiction is in need of further study. Internet addiction follows a trajectory similar to substance-related addictions, as well as gambling and gaming disorders.[9,84] Although Griffiths[9] points to the symptoms traditionally associated with an Internet addiction (salience, mood modification, tolerance, withdrawal, conflict, and relapse), Kuss and Griffiths[67–69] also suggest there is an abundance of neurobiological evidence suggesting its addictive properties. Problematic Internet Use, Internet Addiction Disorder, or Internet Addiction (IA) is characterized by excessive preoccupation, urges, and/or behaviors that ultimately lead to significant impairment and negative consequences.[95]

Several researchers contend that rather than looking at IA per se, an emphasis and focus should be on the specific type of Internet activities in which the individual is engaged (eg, online gambling, gaming disorders, smartphone use) that may prompt them to become addicted.[84,96] For example, studies examining the use of social networking applications, including online chatting,[97,98] and social networking sites,[64,99] have been reported to be highly associated with IA.[84]

Prevalence of Internet Addiction

Although no current "gold standard" measure exists for identifying IA, international prevalence rates of IA have varied considerably, ranging from 1.5% to 8.2%.[100] These rates are dependent on the ages of individuals being assessed as well as geographic differences.[101–103] Given the popularity and widespread accessibility of the Internet, a large number of studies have been conducted among adolescents[104] and university students.[66,84,105] Kuss and colleagues[84] attribute high rates of Internet use among children and adolescents to their unlimited Internet access, flexible schedules, and expectations by teachers and peers that they make use of technology. Studies of youth appear to indicate extremely high prevalence rates of Facebook and Twitter use, with a large percentage of youth indicating an inability to stop using social networking sites and frequently spending excessive amounts of time on these sites.[106] Whether used for gaming or social networking sites, Internet use enables adolescents to stay "connected" with their peers and thus remains highly socially acceptable and desirable to youth.

The fact that IA has been associated with aggression,[107,108] introversion,[107] high sensation seeking,[108] social inhibition,[109] neuroticism,[110,111] lower scores on measures of extroversion,[112] depression and depressive mood disorders,[113,114] anxiety,[115] emotional stability,[116] conduct disorders,[117] general mental health disorders,[118] poor coping strategies, difficulties in school and at home,[119] and the need for psychological escape from their current reality,[120] all point to the potential seriousness of the problem.[10,84] There is a growing body of literature suggesting that Internet-addicted adolescents suffer loss of control, have a poor self-image, low self-esteem, experience social withdrawal, and report familial conflicts.[121] Studies have revealed that under extreme circumstances, a severe IA can lead to dysthymia; bipolar, affective social-anxiety disorders; and major depression.[121] Excessive Internet use has been associated with impaired sleep and eating disorders.[122]

Assessment of Internet Addiction

Diagnosing IA can be challenging.[122] As previously indicated, there are no "gold standard" assessment instruments. Many of the scales developed have been based on the DSM clinical criteria for substance dependence or a gambling disorder (assessing preoccupation, the need to increase the behavior, efforts to control the behavior, emotional responses when trying to reduce or stop Internet use, lying to family members about time spent on the Internet, the use of the Internet to reduce a dysphoric mood, the continuous need for increased use, and negative consequences associated with excessive Internet use). Examples of such scales include the Internet Addiction Diagnostic Questionnaire,[123] the Problematic Internet Use Questionnaire developed by Demetrovics and colleagues,[124] and the Compulsive Internet Use Scale.[125]

THE AGE OF SMARTPHONES

Today's smartphones are part mini-computer and part cell phone. Connected to the Internet, they allow individuals to communicate with anyone; search for information; check email or Facebook messages; play games; do banking; order goods; watch favorite movies, sports, or television shows; and easily find directions.[126] In addition, in recent years there has been an explosion in the number of applications (apps) developed for smartphones, enabling users to do anything from monitoring their health to controlling environmental conditions (eg, alarm, lights, heating/cooling schedules) in their homes.

The number of smartphone users is nearing 2.5 billion in 2019,[127] with analysts projecting more than 6 billion smartphones being in use by 2020.[128] Although user growth is expected to level off in developing markets (ie, North America and Europe), the exponential growth will be led by penetration in less mature markets (ie, Africa, the Middle East).[129]

Youth and Smartphones

In the United States, smartphone ownership has become a nearly ubiquitous element of teen life, with 95% of teens reporting they have a smartphone or access to one, representing a 22% increase from 2014.[130] Smartphone ownership is nearly universal in North America and parts of Europe and Asia, independent of gender, race, ethnicity, and socioeconomic background.[130] Although Internet and smartphone use is on the rise, geographic differences have been noted. A large-scale study in 2014 across Europe (Belgium, Denmark, Ireland, Italy, Portugal, Romania, United Kingdom) revealed that 46% of children ages 9 to 16 years reported owning a smartphone.[131] In South Korea, 84% of individuals older than 3 were found to use a smartphone, with approximately 96% of teenagers reporting smartphone usage,[132] in the United Kingdom, 46% of 9-year-olds own a smartphone and 93% of youth aged 15 own one,[133] and in Switzerland, nearly all adolescents aged 12 to 19 (98%) own a mobile phone (97% of which are smartphones).[134] Although these prevalence studies are not directly comparable given they were conducted over different time periods and use different-age populations, they clearly indicate a growing number of children and adolescents possess or have access to a smartphone. The most commonly reported reason for parents initially giving their children a smartphone is to facilitate contact (either from parent to child or child to parent).[135] In the United States and Japan, youth spend most of the time on their mobile device playing games, watching videos, accessing social networking sites, and messaging.[136,137] Interestingly, individuals (American) between 18 and 24 years old send and receive an average of 2022 texts per month,[138] with texting surpassing voice calls and emails as the most common means of transmitting information, particularly for adolescents and young adults.[139] Whether using one's smartphone for texting, tweeting, sexting, or using social media communications, the prevalence and appeal are overwhelming.

Smartphone Addiction

Similar to excessive gambling, gaming, and Internet use, excessive smartphone use can have adverse mental and physical health consequences. The Pew Research

Center[130] reported that 45% of US teens indicate they are online "almost constantly," and this figure has nearly doubled from 24% in their 2014 to 2015 survey. Youth sleep with their smartphones, eat with their smartphones at their side, and repeatedly check for messages and texts. International research shows similar upward trends in usage. Among Korean youth (aged 11–12), research has revealed they spend, on average, 5.4 hours daily on their smartphones.[140] Although some studies reported a predominance of female individuals addicted to their smartphone, others have revealed greater use and problems among male individuals.[141] Internationally, smartphone addiction prevalence rates among youth have been reported to be 19.9% in Switzerland,[142] 30.9% in South Korea,[143] 10.0% in the United Kingdom,[144] and 6.4% in Turkey.[145] The wide variability in prevalence rates is attributable to the use of different scales and methodologies for measurement.[146,147]

Risks Associated with Excessive Smartphone Use

Despite the many advantages associated with smartphone use (eg, communication, ability to immediately access information, social networking), its increasing popularity and overuse by children and adolescents has resulted in multiple problems.[126] The consequences of excessive smartphone use include depression, anxiety, impulsivity, poor self-regulation, academic difficulties, reduced social interaction, and a lack of familial interaction.[145,148–158] Increased time spent on smartphones also has been shown to be related to lower physical activity and more sedentary behavior, sleep disturbances, and a number of physical problems (neck stiffness, blurred vision, wrist or back pain), and fewer leisure pursuits, such as reading or creating art or music.[126,142,154,159]

Assessing Smartphone Addiction

There are a limited number of instruments for assessing potential smartphone addiction among children and adolescents.[144] Several of the scales in current use include the Smartphone Addiction Scale,[160] Cellular Phone Dependence Questionnaire,[161] and Problematic Mobile Phone Use Questionnaire (PMPUQ)[153] and its short version (PMPUQ-SV).[153] The 27-item Mobile Phone Problem Use Scale (MPPUS) of Bianchi and Phillips[162] is among the most widely used with adults, and has been adapted for use with adolescents (MPPUSA, a 26-item scale).[144]

TREATING GAMBLING, INTERNET, GAMING, AND SMARTPHONE ADDICTIONS

Although it is beyond the scope of this article to go into depth concerning the treatment of behavioral disorders, it is important to note that few children and adolescents voluntarily seek treatment for any of the behavioral disorders discussed. Issues related to abstinence versus controlled use still remain. Although one could argue for abstinence in gambling (especially for children and adolescents), it is difficult to make this argument for Internet or smartphone use. In some jurisdictions, in-patient treatment is growing, especially for individuals with a gaming addiction. Some schools are now requiring children to place their smartphones in their locker at the beginning of the school day and retrieve them only at the end of the day[163]; and governments around the world are trying to develop more effective systems for prohibiting underage youth from gambling. Traditional forms of treatment for several behavioral disorders include cognitive/cognitive behavioral therapy, motivational interviewing, family therapy, and a growing number of online forums and support groups. Yau and colleagues[164] suggest that a comprehensive treatment program for behavioral addictions may want to use an integrated treatment approach, drawing on several different therapeutic approaches that focus on addressing symptoms, as well as the underlying dynamics that contribute to the addictive behavior. Although Yau and colleagues[164] were discussing treatment of a food addiction, this model would be beneficial in working with youth experiencing other forms of behavioral addictions.

Parents play an essential role in helping both prevent and modify their children's behavioral addictions. There is little doubt about the social acceptance of many of the behaviors discussed, and there is ample evidence that children are increasingly being exposed to gambling, gaming, the Internet, and use of mobile technologies earlier and earlier.[165] Gaming, the Internet, and smartphones are commonly used as forms of entertainment and communication. They are also used by parents as a way of keeping their children occupied. The issue remains as to when casual use or engagement becomes problematic. There is considerable evidence that parents remain unaware of the extent to which children engage in these behaviors until they become problematic. Much of this behavior is often modeled on parental behavior. Parents should be encouraged to set limits early on, model appropriate behavior, recognize the warning signs as to when a behavior becomes problematic, and to modify and/or curb excessive use. Time limitations for Internet use, gaming, and smartphone use are often dependent on the age of the individual, the free time available and whether the behavior is interfering with social interactions and school performance. There exists an enormous wealth of knowledge via the Internet concerning strategies to help curb excessive problematic behaviors. There are also a growing number of pediatricians, psychologists, and psychiatrists with clinical expertise to help children and parents.

SUMMARY

Today's youth face different stressors than any generation before them. Not only are they dealing with physiologic changes, increasing academic demands, social pressures, and a difficult employment market, they are doing this in front of an online audience. Youth are expected to be "on" 24 hours a day, 7 days a week. Although technology has made certain tasks easier, the social pressures placed on our teens has increased exponentially. Suicide rates have increased for children younger than 15, and dramatically jumped for youth between age 15 and 24.[166] Based on the 2017 Youth Risk Behaviors Survey, 7.4% of youth in grades 9 to 12 (ages 12–17) reported having made at least one suicide attempt during the past 12 months (2.4% of youth required medical treatment).[166] Although it is impossible to draw a causal link with many of the behavioral disorders discussed, the psychosocial stresses placed on youth resulting from any of the behaviors discussed certainly leads to a wide variety of mental health issues.

There is little doubt that the behavioral addictions discussed (gambling disorders, gaming disorders, IA disorders, and smartphone problems) often develop during childhood and adolescence. Today's youth are not only "connected," but fear they will miss something important when not connected. The excessive use of "screen time" has led to major confrontations with parents over their devices. Awareness of these disorders is essential. Setting limits by parents often results in more conflict. Tracking the amount of screen time children use can provide parents with a better picture of the severity of the problem. Other behavioral disorders, such as gambling, are often more difficult to observe.

Although, with time, some youth may outgrow these disorders as they become adults through a process of natural recovery or, in some cases, through psychological or psychiatric interventions (there is evidence that adult prevalence rates for many of these behavioral disorders are lower compared with adolescents), their consequences and harms may be severe. It is important to recognize that concomitant mental health, academic, social, familial, and interpersonal issues may have longstanding consequences. Although many of the treatment approaches have evolved from work in substance abuse, each disorder requires an understanding of the motivations underlying the behaviors to determine whether abstinence or controlled behavior may be feasible. Although abstinence from gambling and gaming behaviors might be possible, use of the Internet and smartphones is essential. Further understanding of the developmental trajectories and the risk and protective factors for each of these behavioral disorders will ultimately enable us to develop more effective prevention and treatment strategies.

REFERENCES

1. Rosenberg K, Feder L. An introduction to behavioral addictions. Behavioral addictions: criteria, evidence and treatment. New York: Elsevier; 2014. p. 1–17.
2. American Psychiatric Association. Diagnostic and statistical manual of mental disorders: DSM-5. Washington, DC: American Psychiatric Publishing; 2013.
3. Grant J, Potenza MN, Weinstein A, et al. Introduction to behavioral addictions. Am J Drug Alcohol Abuse 2010;36(5):233–41.
4. Rosenberg K, Feder L, editors. Behavioral addictions: criteria, evidence, and treatment. New York: Elsevier; 2014.
5. Petry NM, editor. Behavioral addictions: DSM-5 and beyond. New York: Oxford University Press; 2016.
6. Young K, De Abreu C. Internet addiction: a handbook and guide to evaluation and treatment. New York: John Wiley & Sons; 2010.
7. World Health Organization. International classification of diseases-eleventh revision (ICD-11). (Switzerland): World Health Organization; 2018.
8. American Society of Addiction Medicine. Public policy statement: definition of addiction. Chevy Chase (MD): American Society of Addiction Medicine; 2011.
9. Griffiths MD. A 'components' model of addiction within a biopsychosocial framework. J Subst Use 2005;10(4):191–7.
10. Derevensky J. Behavioral addictions: some developmental consideration. Curr Addict Rep 2019;6(3):313–22.
11. Jessor R, editor. New perspectives on adolescent risk behavior. New York: Cambridge University Press; 1998.
12. Derevensky J. Teen gambling: understanding a growing epidemic. New York: Rowman & Littlefield Publishers; 2012.
13. Jessor R, Van Den Bos J, Vaderryn J, et al. Protective factors in adolescent problem behavior: moderator effects and developmental change. Dev Psychol 1995;31(6):923–33.
14. Dickson L, Derevensky JL, Gupta R. Youth gambling problems: examining risk and protective factors. Int Gamb Stud 2008;8(1):25–47.
15. Jacobs DF. A general theory of addictions: a new theoretical model. J Gambl Behav 1986;2(1):15–31.
16. Calado F, Alexandre J, Griffiths MD. Prevalence of adolescent problem gambling: a systematic review of recent research. J Gambl Stud 2017;33(2):397–424.
17. Volberg R, Gupta R, Griffiths MD, et al. An international perspective on youth gambling prevalence studies. Int J Adolesc Med Health 2010;22:3–38.

18. Gupta R, Derevensky J. Adolescents with gambling problems: from research to treatment. J Gambl Stud 2000;(16):315–42.
19. Andrie E, Tzavara C, Tzavela E, et al. Gambling involvement and problem gambling correlates among European adolescents: results from the EU NET ADB study. Soc Psychiatry Psychiatr Epidemiol 2019. [Epub ahead of print].
20. Hayer T, Griffiths MD. The prevention and treatment of problem gambling in adolescence. In: Gullotta T, Adams G, editors. Handbook of adolescent behavioural problems: evidence-based approaches to prevention and treatment. New York: Springer; 2014. p. 467–86.
21. Jacobs DF. Juvenile gambling in North America: an analysis of long-term trends and future prospects. J Gambl Stud 2000;(16):119–52.
22. Jacobs DF. Youth gambling in North America: long-term trends and future prospects. In: Derevensky J, Gupta R, editors. Gambling problems in youth: theoretical and applied perspectives. New York: Kluwer Academic/Plemun Publishers; 2004.
23. Derevensky J, Gupta R. Prevalence estimates of adolescent gambling: a comparison of the SOGS-RA, DSM-IV-J, and the GA 20 Questions. J Gambl Stud 2000;16:227–51.
24. Campbell C, Derevensky J, Meerkamper E, et al. Parents' perceptions of adolescent gambling: a Canadian national study. J Gamb Iss 2011;25:36–53.
25. Derevensky J, St-Pierre R, Temcheff C, et al. Teacher awareness and attitudes regarding adolescent risky behaviours: is adolescent gambling perceived to be a problem? J Gambl Stud 2014;30:435–51.
26. Sansanwal R, Derevensky J, Lupu I, et al. Knowledge and attitudes regarding adolescent problem gambling: a cross-cultural comparative analysis of Romanian and Canadian teachers. Int J Ment Health Addict 2015;13(1):33–48.
27. Sansanwal R, Derevensky J, Gavriel-Fried B. What mental health professionals in Israel know and think about adolescent problem gambling. Int Gamb Stud 2016;16:67–84.
28. Temcheff C, Derevensky J, St-Pierre R, et al. Beliefs and attitudes of mental health professionals with respect to gambling and other high risk behaviors in schools. Int J Ment Health Addict 2014;12:716–29.
29. Griffiths MD, Parke J. Adolescent gambling on the Internet: a review. Int J Adolesc Med Health 2010;22:59–75.
30. Delfabbro P, King D, Griffiths MD. From adolescent to adult gambling: an analysis of longitudinal gambling patterns in South Australia. J Gambl Stud 2014;30(3):547–63.
31. Productivity Commission. Gambling productivity inquiry report. Melbourne (Australia): Australian Government; 2010.
32. Gupta R, Derevensky J. Familial and social influences on juvenile gambling. J Gambl Stud 1997;13:179–92.
33. Stinchfield R, Winters KC. Gambling and problem gambling among youth. Ann Am Acad Pol Soc Sci 1998;556:172–85.
34. Wallisch LS. Gambling in Texas: 1995 Surveys of adult and adolescent gambling behavior, Executive Summary. Austin (TX): Texas Commission on Alcohol & Drug Abuse; 1996.
35. Hardoon K, Derevensky J, Gutpa R. An examination of the influence of familial, emotional, conduct and cognitive problems, and hyperactivity upon youth risk-taking and adolescent gambling problems. Ontario (Canada): Ontario Problem Gambling Research Center; 2002.

36. Ste-Marie C, Gutpa R, Derevensky J. Anxiety and social stress related to adolescent gambling behavior and substance use. J Child Adolesc Subst Abuse 2006; 16(4):55–74.

37. Dussault F, Brendgen M, Vitaro F, et al. Longitudinal links between impulsivity, gambling problems and depressive symptoms: a transactional model from adolescence to early adulthood. J Child Psychol Psychiatry 2011;52(2):130–8.

38. Gupta R, Derevensky J. An empirical examination of Jacobs' General Theory of Addictions: do adolescent gamblers fit the theory? J Gambl Stud 1998;14: 17–49.

39. Gupta R, Derevensky J. Adolescent gambling behaviour: a prevalence study and examination of the correlates associated with problem gambling. J Gambl Stud 1998;14:319–45.

40. Nower L, Gupta R, Blaszczynski A, et al. Suicidality and depression among youth gamblers: a preliminary examination of three studies. Int Gamb Stud 2004;4(1):70–80.

41. Welte JW, Barnes GM, Tidwell MC, et al. Association between problem gambling and conduct disorder in a national survey of adolescents and young adults in the United States. J Adolesc Health 2009;45(4):396–401.

42. Derevensky J, Gupta R. Adolescents with gambling problems: a synopsis of our current knowledge. J Gamb Iss 2004;10.

43. Gupta R, Derevensky J, Marget N. Coping strategies employed by adolescents with gambling problems. J Child Adolesc Ment Health 2004;9(3):115–20.

44. Lussier I, Derevensky J, Gupta R, et al. Youth gambling behaviors: an examination of the role of resilience. Psychol Addict Behav 2007;21:165–73.

45. Lussier I, Derevensky J, Gupta R, et al. Risk, compensatory, protective, and vulnerability factors related to youth gambling problems. Psychol Addict Behav 2014;28(2):404–13.

46. Bergevin T, Derevensky J, Gupta R, et al. Adolescent gambling: understanding the role of stress and coping. J Gambl Stud 2006;22(2):195–208.

47. Winters KC, Stinchfield RD, Fulkerson J. Toward the development of an adolescent gambling problem severity scale. J Gambl Stud 1993;9:63–84.

48. Fisher S. Measuring pathological gambling in children: The case of fruit machines in the U. K. J Gambl Stud 1992;8:263–85.

49. Fisher S. Developing the DSM-IV-MR-J criteria to identify adolescent problem gambling in non-clinical populations. J Gambl Stud 2000;(16):253–73.

50. Shaffer HJ, LaBrie R, Scanlen KM, et al. Pathological gambling among adolescents: Massachusetts Gambling Screen (MAGS). J Gambl Stud 1994;10: 339–62.

51. Tremblay J, Wiebe J, Stinchfield R, et al. Canadian Adolescent Gambling Inventory (CAGI). Report to the Canadian Centre on Substance Abuse and the Interprovincial Consortium on Gambling Research; Toronto, Ontario, 2015.

52. Derevensky J, Gainsbury S. Social casino gaming and adolescents: should we be concerned and is regulation in sight? Int J Law Psychiatry 2016;44:1–6.

53. Kim H, Hollingshead S, Wohl M. Who spends money to play for free? Identifying who makes micro-transactions on social casino games (and why). J Gambl Stud 2017;33(2):525–38.

54. Kim H, Wohl M, Gupta R, et al. Why do young adults gamble online? A qualitative study of motivations to transition from social casino games to online gambling. Asian J Gambl Issues Public Health 2017;7(1):6.

55. Kim H. Social casino games: current evidence and future directions. Ottawa (Canada): Carleton University; 2017.

56. King D. Online gaming and gambling in children and adolescents—normalising gambling in cyber places: a review of the literature. Melbourne (Australia): University of Adelaide; 2018.

57. McBride J, Derevensky J. Internet gambling and risk-taking among students: an exploratory study. J Behav Addict 2012;1(2):50–8.

58. Marchica L, Derevensky J. Fantasy sports: a growing concern among college student-athletes. Int J Ment Health Addict 2016;14(5):635–45.

59. Gentile D. Pathological video-game use among youth ages 8 to 18: a national study. Psychol Sci 2009;20(5):594–602.

60. Anderson C, Gentile D, Buckley K. Violent video game effects on children and adolescents: theory, research, and public policy. New York: Oxford University Press; 2007.

61. Király O, Nagygyörgy K, Griffiths MD, et al. Problematic online gaming. In: Rosenberg KP, Feder L, editors. Behavioral addictions: criteria, evidence and treatment. New York: Elsevier; 2014. p. 61–97.

62. Newzoo. Newzoo's 2017 report: Insights into the $108.9 billion global games market. 2017. Available at: https://newzoo.com/insights/articles/newzoo-2017-report-insights-into-the-108-9-billion-global-games-market/. Accessed February 5, 2019.

63. Ryan RM, Rigby CS, Przybylski A. The motivational pull of video games: a self-determination theory approach. Motiv Emot 2006;30(4):347–63.

64. Kuss D, Griffiths MD. Online social networking and addiction: a review of the psychological literature. Int J Environ Res Public Health 2011;8(9):3528–52.

65. Rehbein F, Kuhn S, Rumpf H, et al. Internet gaming disorder: a new behavioral addiction. In: Petry NM, editor. Behavioral addictions: DSM-5 and beyond. New York: Oxford University Press; 2016. p. 43–70.

66. Fortson B, Scotti J, Chen Y, et al. Internet use, abuse, and dependence among students at a Southeastern regional university. J Am Coll Health 2007;56(2): 137–44.

67. Kuss D, Griffiths MD. Internet and gaming addiction: a systematic literature review of neuroimaging studies. Brain Sci 2012;2(3):347–74.

68. Kuss D, Griffiths MD. Online gaming addiction in children and adolescents: a review of empirical research. J Behav Addict 2012;1(1):3–22.

69. Kuss D, Griffiths MD. Internet gaming addiction: a systematic review of empirical research. Int J Ment Health Addict 2012;10(2):278–96.

70. Rehbein F, Staudt A, Hanslmaier M, et al. Video game playing in the general adult population of Germany: can higher gaming time of males be explained by gender specific genre preferences? Comput Hum Behav 2016;55:729–35.

71. Eichenbaum A, Kattner F, Bradford D, et al. Role-playing and real-time strategy games associated with greater probability of Internet gaming disorder. Cyberpsychol Behav Soc Netw 2015;18(8):480–5.

72. Lemmens JS, Hendriks SJF. Addictive online games: examining the relationship between game genres and Internet gaming disorder. Cyberpsychol Behav Soc Netw 2016;19(4):270–6.

73. Donati MA, Chiesi F, Ammannato G, et al. Versatility and addiction in gaming: the number of video-game genres played is associated with pathological gaming in male adolescents. Cyberpsychol Behav Soc Netw 2015;18(2): 129–32.

74. Mößle T, Rehbein F. Predictors of problematic video game usage in childhood and adolescence. Sucht 2013;59(3):153–64.

75. Gentile D, Choo H, Liau A, et al. Pathological video game use among youths: a two-year longitudinal study. Pediatrics 2011;127:319–29.

76. Rumpf H, Vermulst A, Kastirke N, et al. Occurence of Internet addiction in a general population sample: a latent class analysis. Eur Addict Res 2014;20(4): 159–66.

77. Mihara S, Higuchi S. Cross-sectional and longitudinal epidemiological studies of Internet gaming disorder: a systematic review of the literature. Psychiatry Clin Neurosci 2017;71(7):425–44.

78. Laconi S, Pirès S, Chabrol H. Internet gaming disorder, motives, game genres and psychopathology. Comput Hum Behav 2017;75:652–9.

79. Rehbein F, Kleimann M, Mößle T. Prevalence and risk factors of video game dependency in adolescence: results of a German nationwide survey. Cyberpsychol Behav Soc Netw 2010;13(3):269–77.

80. Krossbakken E, Torsheim T, Mentzoni RA, et al. The effectiveness of a parental guide for prevention of problematic video gaming in children: a public health randomized controlled intervention study. J Behav Addict 2018;7(1):52–61.

81. King DL, Herd MCE, Delfabbro PH. Motivational components of tolerance in Internet gaming disorder. Comput Hum Behav 2018;78:133–41.

82. King DL, Delfabbro PH, Zwaans T, et al. Clinical features and axis I comorbidity of Australian adolescent pathological Internet and video game users. Aust N Z J Psychiatry 2013;47(11):1058–67.

83. Gentile D, Li D, Khoo A, et al. Mediators and moderators of long-term effects of violent video games on aggressive behavior: practice, thinking, and action. JAMA Pediatr 2014;168(5):450–7.

84. Kuss D, Griffiths MD, Binder J. Internet addiction in students: prevalence and risk factors. Comput Hum Behav 2013;29(3):959–66.

85. King D, Delfabbro PH, Griffiths MD. Video game structural characteristics: a new psychological taxonomy. Int J Ment Health Addict 2010;8(1):90–106.

86. Flaherty C. Cutting academic programs, spending on esports. 2018. Available at: https://www.insidehighered.com/quicktakes/2018/08/20/cutting-academic-programs-spending-esports. Accessed February 3, 2019.

87. Bauer-Wolf J. Video games as a college sport. 2017. Available at: https://www.insidehighered.com/news/2017/06/09/esports-quickly-expanding-colleges. Accessed February 22, 2019.

88. Smith N. eSports catching fire at Ohio State. Washington Post 2018.

89. Igelman A. eSports and Casinos. Available at: https://ggbnews.com/article/esports-and-casinos/2018. Accessed February 12, 2019.

90. Petry NM, Rehbein F, Gentile D, et al. An international consensus for assessing Internet gaming disorder using the new DSM-5 approach. Addiction 2014; 109(9):1399–406.

91. Pontes HM, Kiraly O, Demetrovics Z, et al. The conceptualisation and measurement of DSM-5 Internet Gaming Disorder: the development of the IGD-20 Test. PLoS One 2014;9(10):e110137.

92. Pontes HM, Griffiths MD. Measuring DSM-5 Internet gaming disorder: development and validation of a short psychometric scale. Comput Hum Behav 2015; 45:137–43.

93. Lemmens J, Valkenburg P, Gentile D. The Internet gaming disorder scale. Psychol Assess 2015;27(2):567–82.

94. Lemmens J, Valkenburg P, Peter J. Development and validation of a game addiction scale for adolescents. Media Psychol 2009;12:77–95.

95. Weinstein A, Feder L, Rosenberg K, et al. Internet addiction disorder: overview and controversies. In: Rosenberg K, Feder L, editors. Behavioral addictions: criteria, evidence and treatment. New York: Elsevier; 2014. p. 99–117.

96. Widyanto L, Griffiths MD. Internet addiction: a critical review. Int J Ment Health Addict 2006;4(1):31–51.

97. Huang Y-R. Identity and intimacy crises and their relationship to Internet dependence among college students. Cyberpsychol Behav 2006;9(5):571–6.

98. Leung L. Net-generation attributes and seductive properties of the Internet as predictors of online activities and Internet addiction. Cyberpsychol Behav 2004;7(3):333–48.

99. Leung L, Lee P. The influences of information literacy, Internet addiction and parenting styles on Internet risks. New Media Soc 2012;14(1):117–36.

100. Petersen K, Weymann N, Schelb Y, et al. Pathological Internet use: epidemiology, diagnostics, co-occurring disorders and treatment. Fortschr Neurol Psychiatr 2009;77(5):263–71.

101. Christakis D, Moreno M, Jelenchick L, et al. Problematic Internet usage in US college students: a pilot study. BMC Med 2011;9(1):77.

102. Poli R, Agrimi E. Internet addiction disorder: prevalence in an Italian student population. Nord J Psychiatry 2012;66(1):55–9.

103. Niemz K, Griffiths MD, Banyard P. Prevalence of pathological Internet use among university students and correlations with self-esteem, the General Health Questionnaire (GHQ), and disinhibition. Cyberpsychol Behav 2005;8(6):562–70.

104. Lam L, Peng Z, Mai J, et al. Factors associated with Internet addiction among adolescents. Cyberpsychol Behav 2009;12(5):551–5.

105. Moreno M, Jelenchick L, Cox E, et al. Problematic Internet use among US youth: a systematic review. Arch Pediatr Adolesc Med 2011;165(9):797–805.

106. Cabral J. Is generation Y addicted to social media? Elon Journal of Undergraduate Research in Communications 2011;2(1):5–13.

107. Caplan S, Williams D, Yee N. Problematic Internet use and psychosocial well-being among MMO players. Comput Hum Behav 2009;25(6):1312–9.

108. Mehroof M, Griffiths MD. Online gaming addiction: the role of sensation seeking, self-control, neuroticism, aggression, state anxiety, and trait anxiety. Cyberpsychol Behav 2010;13(3):313–6.

109. Porter G, Starcevic V, Berle D, et al. Recognizing problem video game use. Aust N Z J Psychiatry 2010;44(2):120–8.

110. Dong G, Wang J, Yang X, et al. Risk personality traits of Internet addiction: a longitudinal study of Internet-addicted Chinese university students. Asia Pac Psychiatry 2013;5(4):316–21.

111. Tsai H, Cheng S, Yeh T, et al. The risk factors of Internet addiction—a survey of university freshmen. Psychiatry Res 2009;167(3):294–9.

112. Van der Aa N, Overbeek G, Engels R, et al. Daily and compulsive Internet use and well-being in adolescence: a diathesis-stress model based on big five personality traits. J Youth Adolesc 2009;38(6):765.

113. Morrison C, Gore H. The relationship between excessive Internet use and depression: a questionnaire-based study of 1,319 young people and adults. Psychopathology 2010;43(2):121–6.

114. Tsitsika A, Critselis E, Louizou A, et al. Determinants of Internet addiction among adolescents: a case-control study. ScientificWorldJournal 2011;11:866–74.

115. Kratzer S, Hegerl U. Is "Internet Addiction" a disorder of its own? A study on subjects with excessive Internet use. Psychiatr Prax 2008;35(2):80–3.

116. Bernardi S, Pallanti S. Internet addiction: a descriptive clinical study focusing on comorbidities and dissociative symptoms. Compr Psychiatry 2009;50(6):510–6.

117. Kormas GS, Critselis E, Janikian M, et al. Risk factors and psychosocial characteristics of potential problematic and problematic Internet use among adolescents: a cross-sectional study. BMC Public Health 2011;11(1):595.

118. Kawabe K, Horiuchi F, Ochi M, et al. Internet addiction: prevalence and relation with mental states in adolescents. Psychiatry Clin Neurosci 2016;70(9):405–12.

119. Milani L, Osualdella D, Di Blasio P. Quality of interpersonal relationships and problematic Internet use in adolescence. Cyberpsychol Behav 2009;12(6):681–4.

120. Kwon J, Chung C, Lee J. The effects of escape from self and interpersonal relationship on the pathological use of Internet games. Community Ment Health J 2011;47(1):113–21.

121. Cerniglia L, Zoratto F, Cimino S, et al. Internet addiction in adolescence: neurobiological, psychosocial and clinical issues. Neurosci Biobehav Rev 2017;76(Pt A):174–84.

122. Young K. Clinical assessment of Internet-addicted clients. In: Young K, Nabuco de Abreu C, editors. Internet addiction. New Jersey: John Wiley & Sons; 2011. p. 19–34.

123. Young KS. Internet addiction: the emergence of a new clinical disorder. Cyber Psychology Behav 1998;1(3):237–44.

124. Demetrovics Z, Szeredi B, Rozsa S. The three-factor model of Internet addiction: the development of the Problematic Internet Use Questionnaire. Behav Res Methods 2008;40(2):563–74.

125. Meerkerk GJ, Van Den Eijnden RJJM, Vermulst AA, et al. The compulsive Internet use scale (CIUS): some psychometric properties. Cyberpsychol Behav 2009;12(1):1–6.

126. Choi SW, Kim DJ, Choi JS, et al. Comparison of risk and protective factors associated with smartphone addiction and Internet addiction. J Behav Addict 2015;4(4):308–14.

127. Statista. Number of smartphone users worldwide from 2014 to 2020 (in billions). 2019. Available at: https://www.statista.com/statistics/330695/number-of-smartphone-users-worldwide/. Accessed February 28, 2019.

128. IHS Markit. More than six billion smartphones by 2020. 2017. Available at: https://news.ihsmarkit.com/press-release/technology/more-six-billion-smartphones-2020-ihs-markit-says. Accessed January 20, 2019.

129. Lunden I. 6.1B smartphone users globally by 2020, Overtaking basic fixed phone subscriptions. 2015. Available at: https://techcrunch.com/2015/06/02/6-1b-smartphone-users-globally-by-2020-overtaking-basic-fixed-phone-subscriptions/. Accessed February 3, 2019.

130. Pew Research Center. Teens, social media & technology 2018. 2018. Available at: http://www.pewinternet.org/2018/05/31/teens-social-media-technology-2018/. Accessed February 5, 2019.

131. Mascheroni G, Ólafsson K. The mobile Internet: access, use, opportunities and divides among European children. New Media Soc 2015;18(8):1657–79.

132. Korea Internet and Security Agency. 2016 survey on Internet usage. Available at: http://www.kisa.or.kr/eng/usefulreport/surveyReport_View.jsp?cPage=1&p_No=262&b_No=262&d_No=80&ST=&SV=; 2018.

133. Statista. Share of children owning tablets and smartphones in the United Kingdom (UK) from 2017, by age. 2017. Available at: https://www.statista.com/statistics/805397/children-ownership-of-tablets-smartphones-by-age-uk/.

134. Willemse I, Waller G, Genner S, et al. JAMES: Jugend, Aktivitäten, Medien – Erhebung Schweiz [JAMES: Youth, Activities, Media– Survey Switzerland]. Zürich (Switzerland): Zürcher Hochschule für angewandte Wissenschaften; 2014.

135. Nielsen. Mobile kids: the parent, the child and the smartphone. 2017. Available at: https://www.nielsen.com/us/en/insights/news/2017/mobile-kids–the-parent-the-child-and-the-smartphone.html.

136. Statista. Minutes spent daily on mobile devices among Japanese teenagers in 2017, by activity and gender. 2017. Available at: https://www.statista.com/statistics/758200/japan-daily-mobile-device-use-teens-by-activity-gender/.

137. Statista. Share of teenage smartphone users in the United States who spent more than 3 hours on selected mobile activities every day as of August 2016. 2016. Available at: https://www.statista.com/statistics/722531/us-teen-mobile-time-spent-activities/.

138. Experian. Young adults: texting is just as meaningful as a phone call. 2012. Available at: http://www.experian.com/blogs/marketing-forward/2012/12/03/young-adults-texting-is-just-as-meaningful-as-a-phone-call/.

139. Newport F. The new era of communication among Americans. Available at: http://www.gallup.com/poll/179288/new-era-communication-americans.aspx.

140. Jeong S-H, Kim H, Yum J-Y, et al. What type of content are smartphone users addicted to? SNS vs. games. Comput Hum Behav 2016;54:10–7.

141. Randler C, Wolfgang L, Matt K, et al. Smartphone addiction proneness in relation to sleep and morningness-eveningness in German adolescents. J Behav Addict 2016;5(3):465–73.

142. Haug S, Castro RP, Kwon M, et al. Smartphone use and smartphone addiction among young people in Switzerland. J Behav Addict 2015;4(4):299–307.

143. Cha SS, Seo BK. Smartphone use and smartphone addiction in middle school students in Korea: prevalence, social networking service, and game use. Health Psychol Open 2018;5(1):1–15.

144. Lopez-Fernandez O, Honrubia-Serrano L, Freixa-Blanxart M, et al. Prevalence of problematic mobile phone use in British adolescents. Cyberpsychol Behav Soc Netw 2014;17(2):91–8.

145. Aker S, Sahin MK, Sezgin S, et al. Psychosocial factors affecting smartphone addiction in university students. J Addict Nurs 2017;28(4):215–9.

146. Lopez-Fernandez O. Short version of the Smartphone Addiction Scale adapted to Spanish and French: towards a cross-cultural research in problematic mobile phone use. Addict Behav 2017;64:275–80.

147. Lopez-Fernandez O, Honrubia-Serrano ML, Freixa-Blanxart M. Spanish adaptation of the "Mobile Phone Problem Use Scale" for adolescent population. Adicciones 2012;24(2):123–30 [in Spanish].

148. Hawi NS, Samaha M. The relations among social media addiction, self-esteem, and life satisfaction in university students. Soc Sci Comput Rev 2016;35(5):576–86.

149. Junco R. In-class multitasking and academic performance. Comput Hum Behav 2012;28(6):2236–43.

150. Junco R, Cotten SR. No A 4 U: The relationship between multitasking and academic performance. Comput Educ 2012;59(2):505–14.

151. Lin Y-H, Chang L-R, Lee Y-H, et al. Development and validation of the Smartphone Addiction Inventory (SPAI). PLoS One 2014;9(6):e98312.

152. Lin Y-H, Chiang C-L, Lin P-H, et al. Proposed diagnostic criteria for smartphone addiction. PLoS One 2016;11(11):e0163010.

153. Billieux J, Van Der Linden M, Rochat L. The role of impulsivity in actual and problematic use of the mobile phone. Appl Cogn Psychol 2008;22(9):1195–210.

154. Lepp A, Li J, Barkley JE, et al. Exploring the relationships between college students' cell phone use, personality and leisure. Comput Hum Behav 2015;43:210–9.

155. Demirci K, Akgonul M, Akpinar A. Relationship of smartphone use severity with sleep quality, depression, and anxiety in university students. J Behav Addict 2015;4(2):85–92.

156. Samaha M, Hawi N. Relationships among smartphone addiction, stress, academic performance, and satisfaction with life. Comput Hum Behav 2016;57:321–5.

157. Panek E, Khang H, Liu Y, et al. Profiles of problematic smartphone users: a comparison of South Korean and US college students. Korea Obs 2018;49(3):437–64.

158. Kim D, Lee Y, Lee J, et al. Development of Korean Smartphone Addiction Proneness Scale for Youth. PLoS One 2014;9(5):e97920.

159. Hwang K, Yoo Y, Cho O. Smartphone overuse and upper extremity pain, anxiety, depression and interpersonal relationships among college students. Journal of the Korea Contents Association 2012;12(10):365–75.

160. Kwon M, Lee J-Y, Won W-Y, et al. Development and validation of a Smartphone Addiction Scale (SAS). PLoS One 2013;8(2).

161. Toda M, Monden K, Kubo K, et al. Cellular phone dependence tendency of female university students. Nihon Eiseigaku Zasshi 2004;59(4):383–6.

162. Bianchi A, Phillips JG. Psychological predictors of problem mobile phone use. Cyberpsychol Behav 2005;8(1):39–51.

163. Smith R. France bans smartphones from schools. 2018. Available at: https://www.cnn.com/2018/07/31/europe/france-smartphones-school-ban-intl/index.html.

164. Yau YH, Gottleib C, Krasna L, et al. Food addiction: evidence, evaluation and treament. In: Rosenberg K, Feder L, editors. Behavioral addictions. New York: Elsevier; 2014. p. 143–84.

165. Chiong C, Shuler C, editors. Learning: is there an app for that. Investigations of young children's usage and learning with mobile devices and apps. New York: The Joan Ganz Cooney Center at Sesame Workshop; 2010.

166. American Foundation for Suicide Prevention. Suicide statistics. 2019. Available at: https://afsp.org/about-suicide/suicide-statistics/.

Contingency Management
Using Incentives to Improve Outcomes for Adolescent Substance Use Disorders

Catherine Stanger, PhD*, Alan J. Budney, PhD

KEYWORDS

- Incentives • Contingency management • Adolescent • Substance use • Treatment
- Review

KEY POINTS

- Contingency management (CM) interventions can increase abstinence among youth with substance use problems.
- In developing CM interventions, it is important to consider target outcomes; objective monitoring; and the timing, magnitude, and type of rewards and consequences.
- Parents can successfully implement CM at home with training and support.

In the past decades, multiple studies testing interventions for adolescent substance use problems have shown that youth in treatment of substance use problems have better outcomes than those not in treatment, and there are multiple interventions that have been identified as well established or probably efficacious.[1] Contingency management (CM) is one such intervention. The CM approach grew out of the disciplines of behavioral pharmacology and behavior analysis that demonstrated substance use can be conceptualized as a learned behavior that is maintained, in part, by pharmacological actions (reinforcing effects) of the substance in conjunction with social and other nonpharmacological reinforcements that occur in the context of substance use. As such, CM capitalizes on knowledge that drug seeking and drug use can be reduced by arranging relevant environmental contingencies, such that incompatible or competing prosocial reinforcing activities are made more available and drug abstinence is directly reinforced while drug use is punished. Typically, CM interventions are used as part of a comprehensive substance use treatment program, including some form of individual or family-based intervention.

This work was supported by NIH Grants DA15186 and P30DA029926. None of the authors has any conflict of interest or other disclosures.

Center for Technology and Behavioral Health, Geisel School of Medicine at Dartmouth, Dartmouth College, 46 Centerra Parkway, EverGreen Center Suite 300, HB 7255, Lebanon, NH 03766, USA

* Corresponding author.

E-mail address: Catherine.stanger@dartmouth.edu

CM programs (1) identify and specifically define target therapeutic behaviors, such as drug abstinence; (2) carefully monitor the target behavior(s) objectively on a prespecified schedule; and (3) deliver reinforcing or punishing events (eg, tangible rewards or incentives and loss of privileges) when the target behavior is or is not achieved. Often CM programs are managed and delivered directly by program staff. In addition, CM interventions for youth often guide parents in developing and implementing a CM program at home. The goals of CM interventions are to systematically weaken the influence of reinforcement derived from substance use and to increase the frequency and magnitude of reinforcement derived from healthier alternative activities, especially those that are incompatible with continued substance use.

PRINCIPLES OF CONTINGENCY MANAGEMENT

CM interventions are defined by the following metrics: the target behavior, the method of monitoring of the target behavior, the schedule used to deliver positive or negative consequences, the type of consequence, and the magnitude of the consequence. The most commonly selected target behavior used in CM programs has been drug abstinence. CM programs, however, also have targeted medication compliance, counseling attendance, and completion of prosocial activities or lifestyle changes. When choosing targets, it is important to be aware that successful change in one behavior may not result in change in another. For example, treatment attendance may improve by providing incentives for coming to sessions, but drug use might not be affected.[2] Thus, it is recommended that, if possible, abstinence should always be a target behavior, although other supplemental behaviors may be targeted as well provided they can be objectively defined and monitored, as described as follows.

Effective monitoring of the targeted behavior is essential to a CM program, because consequences (reinforcement or punishment) must be applied systematically in order to be effective. When abstinence is the target behavior, this typically involves some form of biochemical verification, usually via urinalysis testing. Such testing requires careful planning so that the schedule of testing (frequency) allows optimal detection of substance use and abstinence. For example, detection windows range from hours (for alcohol use) to many days (cannabis) and depend on the type of testing used (eg, breath, urine, and saliva). The importance of having a method for objectively and reliably verifying whether a target behavior occurred pertains as well to other target behaviors (eg, attending self-help meeting, going to the gym, attending an after-school program, and completing therapeutic practice assignments). Reliance on self-reports of drug use or completion of other therapeutic tasks is not adequate for effective delivery of a CM program.

The schedule of reinforcement or punishment refers to the temporal relation between the target behavior and the delivery of the consequence. Generally, efficacy is likely to improve as the temporal delay between the occurrence of the target behavior and delivery of the consequence decreases. For example, all else being equal, providing positive reinforcement for drug abstinence on the same day on which a youth submits a negative urine specimen likely is more effective than waiting a week before reinforcement is delivered. For this reason, the use of rapid drug tests in the clinic setting is preferred over laboratory tests that do not provide immediate results because they permit more immediate reinforcement of abstinence. In working with clinicians and researchers in diverse settings who are interested in using CM with their clients or patients, questions often arise about the need for and implementation of urine drug testing. Although it can be challenging to address positive urine drug test results in real time, it may help to think of such information as similar to many other health status indicators collected during a health visit that can guide the clinical interaction (eg, weight, blood pressure, and hemoglobin A_{1c}). Objective information about substance use is not only the most important target for CM but also a vital marker of problem severity and response to intervention.

Schedules with frequent opportunities for reinforcement (eg, at least weekly) are more likely to engender and strengthen abstinence. Once a behavior is established, less frequent schedules typically are considered for maintenance of behavior change. One schedule that has demonstrated efficacy across multiple substance abuse treatment studies is a fixed schedule with escalating rewards and a reset contingency (typically referred to as abstinence-based vouchers or incentives[3]). This schedule provides monetary rewards for each negative sample that can be held in a clinic account or loaded onto a reloadable credit card, with a small (usually financial) reward for the first negative sample and rewards increasing in value with each subsequent negative sample. Positive samples reset the reward value to the starting point, but a period of abstinence can reset the value back to the prior maximum. In addition, rewards can be provided according to an intermittent schedule using the fishbowl method,[4] in which negative samples earn the opportunity to complete draws that have a possibility of winning a reward, with rewards of varying values available.

The magnitude of reinforcement is also an important factor that can greatly affect the efficacy of CM interventions. For example, if the goal is drug abstinence, a $10 incentive for each negative drug test is likely to be more effective in increasing abstinence than an incentive worth $2.00. Multiple studies have demonstrated that greater magnitude schedules of reinforcement have resulted in better abstinence outcomes than lower magnitude.[5]

The type of reinforcers or punishers used in a CM program also can be critical to its success. Individuals vary greatly in terms of the types of goods and services that they value and hence that will serve as effective reinforcers/incentives. For example, a specific reinforcer (eg, pizza or movie theater passes) that serves as an effective incentive for one youth may not be reinforcing for another. Use of a range of incentives or allowing youth to choose their incentive can increase the probability that the incentive will be effective and facilitate the desired target behavior. Gift cards or reloadable credit cards often are used because they serve as flexible rewards, allowing youth to select personalized rewards that vary over time.

There are excellent resources available to assist clinicians and researchers in developing CM interventions. Examples include a National Institute on Drug Abuse and Substance Abuse and Mental Health Services Administration Blending Initiative, Promoting Awareness of Motivational Incentives,[6] online information and training (https://arenaebp.com/), and published manuals.[7,8]

RESEARCH ON CONTINGENCY MANAGEMENT WITH YOUTH

In 2 prior articles, the authors reviewed research on CM for substance use among youth prior to 2010[9] and from 2010 to 2016.[10] Since the publication of the latter article, the authors have become aware of 2 additional studies using CM with adolescents.[11,12] Most of these studies have involved youth whose primary or most frequent substance used is cannabis and have demonstrated efficacy of CM across highly diverse settings (school, clinic, juvenile justice, and continuing care), platform interventions using fixed (ie, vouchers) and intermittent (ie, fishbowl) incentive schedules, and incentive magnitude (approximately $25 to $725 total/ approximately $6 to $50 per week).

These studies fall into several distinct categories. First, there is a group of studies that used CM to target tobacco use among high school students.[13–16] Most of these studies were conducted in the school setting, but some also have been implemented remotely.[15,16] Across studies, 4-week abstinence rates generally were greater than 50%. One study also used a similar CM model to target substance use (primarily cannabis use) in the school setting, comparing brief motivational interviewing plus CM to brief motivational interviewing alone.[17] Results indicated greater reductions in cannabis use days per month when CM was added to motivational interviewing, with significant differences between conditions at the end of the 8-week intervention period but not at the 16-week follow-up assessment.

A series of studies has tested integration of family-based CM with juvenile drug court.[18] Incentives for abstinence were provided by both the clinic and parents, who also received instruction in setting up a home-based CM program. Youth receiving CM had decreased odds of a cannabis-positive urine test throughout the 9-month intervention (ie, documenting cannabis use) relative to control group youth who received drug court as usual. At the 9-month assessment, 20% of the youth in the CM condition versus 34% of the control youth tested positive for cannabis. This program has an excellent manual available[8] and is widely disseminated.[19]

CM also has been tested for adolescents stepping down from residential substance use treatment.[20] Youth receiving CM had more days of abstinence from cannabis through the 9-month post-treatment follow-up compared with usual continuing care.

The authors have conducted a series of 3 randomized clinical trials testing the impact of CM when added to an evidence-based individual counseling platform.[11,21,22] This 14-week CM intervention integrates clinic-delivered incentives (approximately $590 maximum for continuous abstinence) with home-based CM, in which parents receive instruction and weekly support in developing and implementing a substance monitoring contract (SMC) that specifies rewards for documented abstinence and consequences for substance use. Parents also earned incentives for session attendance and compliance with the SMC (maximum earnings approximately $270).

The home-based SMC specifies positive and negative consequences to be delivered by the parents in response to documented abstinence or use (based on clinic based urine drug test results) (**Fig. 1**). The consequences are determined via a collaborative process between therapist, parent, and adolescent and are revaluated each week during weekly counseling sessions. This contract uses the same target (abstinence), schedule (at least weekly), and monitoring method (urine drug testing) as the authors' clinic-based CM. Parents also are provided with disposable breathalyzers to test for alcohol use at home (see handout in **Fig. 2**). Parents personalize the type of consequence (monetary, voucher type system, or privileges) and the magnitude of the consequences, and these factors change throughout treatment in response to treatment success or failure. Examples of rewards have included earning a prespecified amount of money for each negative sample, family activities like going out to dinner or choosing the menu for dinner at home, and access to the family car or gas money. Examples of consequences have included restrictions on media/Internet/gaming/or phone use, grounding, and extra household chores. The procedures for working with parents to establish and implement their home contract were based on Adolescent Transitions,[23] an evidence-based parent training intervention. This model is now known as the Family Check-Up (https://reachinstitute.asu.edu/family-check-up), and diverse training options for providers plus information for families are available.

Clinicians sometimes raise concerns about how parents might respond to test results indicating drug use. Working with parents to develop a home SMC can reduce conflict about test results, because parents and teens will have established a plan in advance for how to respond to the results—positive or negative. Moreover, reminders that the primary purpose of testing is to provide teens with an opportunity to

Substance Monitoring Contract

If _____'s urine drug screen is negative (no drugs detected or reported) and there were no positive or refused alcohol breath tests since the last drug screen, I will:

1. Praise their progress!
2. Ask how I can help them keep up the good work.
3. Celebrate their progress by:

    _____
    _____
    _____

If _____'s urine drug screen is positive (drugs detected or reported) and/or there were positive or refused alcohol breath tests since the last drug screen, and/or the urine screen is refused, I will:

1. Remain calm!
2. Not give a lecture
3. Ask how I can help them
4. Express confidence that they can do better next time
5. Use the following consequence:

    _____

_____
Parent Signature   Date

_____
Teen Signature   Date

_____
Therapist Signature   Date

Fig. 1. Substance monitoring contract for home-based contingency management.

demonstrate that they are abstinent and to earn rewards and privileges can help maintain a positive attitude toward the SMC and testing in general. Persistent positive test results indicating persistent substance use suggest the need for a higher level of care. **Fig. 3** provides a sample handout the authors have used with teens and parents to provide a rationale for and information about the urine monitoring program. If clinic-based urine testing is not available, parents can consider implementing these procedures at home, although the authors strongly recommend clinician support in implementing such a procedure because it has many challenges.

Across the 3 randomized clinical trials, there were consistent positive effects of CM during treatment. For example, in the first study,[22] CM enhanced continuous abstinence outcomes, engendering more weeks of continuous cannabis abstinence during treatment. More participants who received CM than those who did not achieve greater than or equal to 8 weeks (53% vs 30%) and greater than or equal to 10 weeks of continuous abstinence (50% vs 19%). There was, however, no significant between-condition difference in abstinence 9 months post-treatment. There was an increase in cannabis use from discharge to 9-month follow-up, that, although not returning to intake levels, was of significant concern. In the second study,[21] youth receiving CM were more likely to achieve 4 weeks of continuous cannabis abstinence during treatment (48%) than were those not receiving CM (30%). In addition, among youth with at least 1 negative urine drug test during treatment, those who received CM had significantly more weeks of continuous abstinence from cannabis than those who did not receive CM. They also were significantly more likely to be abstinent at the end of treatment, but rates of abstinence were comparable between conditions at post-treatment follow-up assessments, and significant relapse was observed. Self-reports of cannabis

Home Alcohol Testing Guidelines and Plan

Most urine drug tests do not test for alcohol use. Parents participating in this program will be given breathalyzers to use at home to tell if their teen has used alcohol recently. We will show you how to use them.

We want you to ask your teen to take the breath test every day, and especially when you think they might have used alcohol.

You should follow these steps:

Ask your teen if they have used alcohol that day.

> **If they say yes**, they used alcohol, you do not need to do the test.
> **If they say no**, they didn't use alcohol, ask them to take the test.
>
>> **If they refuse to take the test**, you should assume they used alcohol and follow the steps below.
>> **If they take the test, and it is negative** [indicates no alcohol use], thank them for taking the test and praise them for not using alcohol.
>> **If they take the test and it is positive** [indicates alcohol use], follow the steps below.

If your teen has used alcohol [breath test is positive, teen refuses to take test, or teen admits use], you should:

> Remain calm, don't yell or lecture
>
> *Not* help your teen get out of trouble [e.g., make excuses for them, protect them from the consequences of using]
>
> Express disappointment once
>
> Do what you need to do to ensure your teen's safety, **such as taking the keys to the car(s) so the teen cannot drive**
>
> Call your therapist the next day
>
> Use the following consequence:_____

Fig. 2. Alcohol testing guidelines and plan for home-based contingency management.

use frequency showed sustained decreases during treatment and post-treatment for all conditions. Thus, the effect of CM was greater when change in cannabis use was assessed as continuous abstinence and measured by urine drug tests than as days of use and measured by self-report. In the authors' most recent CM study,[11] which focused on youth with alcohol use problems with or without comorbid cannabis use, a similar percentage of youth maintained complete alcohol abstinence across the 36-week follow-up in both conditions. Among youth not entirely abstinent from alcohol, however, those receiving CM reported fewer alcohol use days during the 36 weeks after the end of treatment than those not receiving CM. Among youth who also used cannabis at baseline, results showed similar benefits of CM on cannabis use days.

PREDICTORS OF CONTINGENCY MANAGEMENT EFFICACY

Across all these studies with youth, no trial has tested the impact of CM magnitude (ie, compared different magnitudes or schedules) for substance using youth. To date, no

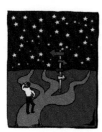

COMMON QUESTIONS ABOUT URINE TESTING

- **Why is urine monitoring an important part of this program?**

  - It helps decrease substance use

  - It keeps the focus of treatment on an important problem (substance use)

  - It gives us and your parents a chance to "catch you" *not* using drugs or alcohol

  - It gives us and your parents a chance to give you incentives, praise, or other kinds of positive support for abstinence

- It can help you and your therapist detect and work on relapse triggers – before use escalates

- It can help you overcome trying to hide substance use because of embarrassment, pride, or not wanting to get into trouble

- It can help you regain credibility with friends, parents, teachers, employers, etc. It can reassure everyone that you continue to do well

Remember - the primary reason for testing is an optimistic one. We want to know that you are not using!

- **WHAT DOES IT MEAN TO TEST "NEGATIVE"?**

  Testing NEGATIVE does not always mean that there is no trace of a substance(s) in your system. It means that you have a low level as a result of not using in the past few days.

- **WHEN I STOP USING DRUGS, HOW SOON WILL I TEST NEGATIVE?**

An average regular marijuana user will test negative after 2 weeks of no use. Other drugs and alcohol clear the body more quickly.

- **AFTER I START TO TEST NEGATIVE FOR MARIJUANA, WILL ALL MY TESTS BE NEGATIVE?**

The "washout period" is when your body is gradually ridding itself of marijuana. Because this "detoxification" can be influenced by your level of physical activity and certain bodily processes, it is possible that you may have a positive test in this period, even though you report not using marijuana, and have had a negative test before. Continue avoiding marijuana and you will see another negative reading at your next visit!

- **WHAT HAPPENS IF I USE MARIJUANA OR USE OTHER DRUGS AFTER TESTING NEGATIVE?**

If you use any marijuana or other drugs, it is likely that you will test positive on your next drug test.

- **PEOPLE SAY THAT THERE ARE METHODS AND PRODUCTS THAT CAN RID MY BODY OF MARIJUANA AND OTHER SUBSTANCES AND MAKE ME HAVE A NEGATIVE DRUG TEST. IS THIS TRUE?**

They don't work and they can be very expensive. Not using drugs is the way to guarantee a negative reading, and it will not empty your wallet.

- **PEOPLE SAY TO DRINK LOTS OF WATER TO GET A NEGATIVE READING, IS THIS TRUE?**

If you drink lots of water, the urine test may indicate that your sample is too dilute and cannot be read. At that point we may ask that you wait at least 4 hours and provide another urine sample within 24 hours. Even if you are not trying to "flush," drinking a lot can cause your urine to be too dilute. If you have a dilute sample on 2 consecutive days, your sample will be considered "positive."

- **IS THERE FOOD I SHOULD AVOID EATING?**

While you are receiving urine testing you should avoid eating poppy seeds. Foods that can contain poppy seeds include bagels, muffins, and other baked goods. Eating poppy seeds may give you an opiate-positive reading. It is your job to take the steps necessary to avoid any substance-positive readings!

- **WHAT DO I DO IF I THINK MY DRUG TEST IS WRONG?**

Please discuss this with your therapist.

Fig. 3. Handout addressing common questions about urine drug testing.

trial has systematically tested the independent or combined efficacy of clinic-based CM versus parent-based CM. The best outcomes across studies were reported for youth with the lowest rates of baseline substance use, that is, those in juvenile drug court or those entering continuing care after residential treatment.[18,20] Intermediate, less enduring outcomes were reported for youth in outpatient and school-based settings.[17,21] Finally, across studies, long-term reduction in use or abstinence among youth remains a serious challenge, even among those who show better post-treatment outcomes. The one study focused on continuing care suggests that including additional targets of CM, such as engagement in specific types of prosocial activities, together with targeting abstinence might better facilitate enduring change.[20]

For the most part, studies have shown that although many baseline characteristics are associated with poorer treatment outcomes (eg, age, gender, ethnicity, and presence of comorbid mental health problems), there are not differential effects of CM across such groups.[18,24] Research is particularly limited, however, on moderation of CM efficacy by cognitive characteristics, such as delay discounting or other constructs related to executive function, including self-regulation or emotion regulation. The authors reported a post hoc analysis showing that youth with disruptive behavior disorder diagnoses (DBDs) in addition to cannabis use disorder had better outcomes when they received CM.[25] DBD-negative adolescents who received abstinence-based CM did not have significantly better cannabis use outcomes compared with counseling only. This may have been due to a ceiling effect; that is, DBD-negative adolescents receiving evidence-based individual counseling had good clinical outcomes, making it more difficult to demonstrate improved outcomes with abstinence-based CM. These findings highlight the importance of future research focused on testing CM and other treatment approaches tailored to pretreatment youth characteristics.

SUMMARY AND FUTURE DIRECTIONS

CM strategies can be effective for retaining youth in treatment, increasing treatment attendance, and promoting abstinence across multiple types of substance use problems. The growing acceptance of abstinence-based CM as one of the most efficacious interventions for youth SUD is evidenced by its recent use as a treatment platform in several clinical trials of new behavioral or pharmacological treatments that seek strategies to further enhance outcomes for adolescents.[26,27] That said, it is critical to attend to the defining components that make up each unique CM intervention, including the target, the monitoring method, the schedule of reinforcement, and the magnitude and type of rewards used, because each can influence intervention efficacy. Fortunately, evidence-based training and manuals are now available to guide research and practice. Avenues for future research include testing the efficacy of a solely parent-administered CM intervention without clinic-delivered CM incentives and developing CM models focused on maintaining treatment gains and preventing relapse. The authors also expect that the growing development and application of diverse technological devices and platforms to improve health behavior should provide a surplus of ideas and innovations for adapting and implementing CM-based programs to better address adolescent substance use problems.[28]

REFERENCES

1. Hogue A, Henderson CE, Becker SJ, et al. Evidence base on outpatient behavioral treatments for adolescent substance use, 2014-2017: outcomes, treatment delivery, and promising horizons. J Clin Child Adolesc Psychol 2018;47(4): 499–526.

2. Iguchi MY, Lamb RJ, Belding MA, et al. Contingent reinforcement of group partic-ipation versus abstinence in a methadone maintenance program. Exp Clin Psy-chopharmacol 1996;4:315–21.
3. Higgins ST, Heil SH, Lussier JP. Clinical implications of reinforcement as a deter-minant of substance use disorders. Annu Rev Psychol 2004;55:431–61.
4. Petry NM, Peirce JM, Stitzer ML, et al. Effect of prize-based incentives on out-comes in stimulant abusers in outpatient psychosocial treatment programs: a na-tional drug abuse treatment clinical trials network study. Arch Gen Psychiatry 2005;62:1148–56.
5. Lussier JP, Heil SH, Mongeon JA, et al. A meta-analysis of voucher-based reinforcement therapy for substance use disorders. Addiction 2006;101(2): 192–203.
6. Hamilton J, Kellogg S, Killeen T, et al. Promoting Awareness of Motivational Incen-tives (PAMI). 2009. Available at: http://pami.nattc.org/explore/priorityareas/science/blendinginitiative/pami/. Accessed September 29, 2009.
7. Petry N. Contingency management for substance abuse treatment: a guide to im-plementing this evidence-based practice. New York: Routledge; 2011.
8. Henggeler SW, Cunningham PB, Rowland MD, et al. Contingency management for adolescent substance abuse: a practitioner's guide. New York: Guilford Press; 2012.
9. Stanger C, Budney AJ. Contingency management approaches for adolescent substance use disorders. Child Adolesc Psychiatr Clin N Am 2010;19(3):547–62.
10. Stanger C, Lansing AH, Budney AJ. Advances in research on contingency man-agement for adolescent substance use. Child Adolesc Psychiatr Clin N Am 2016; 25(4):645–59.
11. Stanger C, Scherer EA, Babbin SF, et al. Abstinence based incentives plus parent training for adolescent alcohol and other substance misuse. Psychol Addict Be-hav 2017;31(4):385–92.
12. Letourneau EJ, McCart MR, Sheidow AJ, et al. First evaluation of a contingency management intervention addressing adolescent substance use and sexual risk behaviors: risk reduction therapy for adolescents. J Subst Abuse Treat 2017;72: 56–65.
13. Cavallo DA, Cooney JL, Duhig AM, et al. Combining cognitive behavioral therapy with contingency management for smoking cessation in adolescent smokers: a preliminary comparison of two different CBT formats. Am J Addict 2007;16(6): 468–74.
14. Krishnan-Sarin S, Cavallo DA, Cooney JL, et al. An exploratory randomized controlled trial of a novel high-school-based smoking cessation intervention for adolescent smokers using abstinence-contingent incentives and cognitive behavioral therapy. Drug Alcohol Depend 2013;132(1–2):346–51.
15. Kong G, Goldberg AL, Dallery J, et al. An open-label pilot study of an intervention using mobile phones to deliver contingency management of tobacco abstinence to high school students. Exp Clin Psychopharmacol 2017;25(5):333–7.
16. Reynolds B, Dallery J, Shroff P, et al. A web-based contingency management program with adolescent smokers. J Appl Behav Anal 2008;41(4):597–601.
17. Stewart DG, Felleman BI, Arger CA. Effectiveness of motivational incentives for adolescent marijuana users in a school-based intervention. J Subst Abuse Treat 2015;58:43–50.
18. Henggeler SW, McCart MR, Cunningham PB, et al. Enhancing the effectiveness of juvenile drug courts by integrating evidence-based principles. J Consult Clin Psychol 2012;80(2):264–75.

19. Cunningham PB, Henggeler SW. The development and transportability of multi-systemic therapy-substance abuse: a treatment for adolescents with substance use disorders AU - Randall, Jeff. J Child Adolesc Subst Abuse 2018;27(2):59–66.

20. Godley MD, Godley SH, Dennis ML, et al. A randomized trial of assertive continuing care and contingency management for adolescents with substance use disorders. J Consult Clin Psychol 2014;82(1):40–51.

21. Stanger C, Ryan SR, Scherer EA, et al. Clinic- and home-based contingency management plus parent training for adolescent cannabis use disorders. J Am Acad Child Adolesc Psychiatry 2015;54(6):445–53.

22. Stanger C, Budney AJ, Kamon JL, et al. A randomized trial of contingency management for adolescent marijuana abuse and dependence. Drug Alcohol Depend 2009;105(3):240–7.

23. Dishion TJ, Kavanagh K. Intervening in adolescent problem behavior: a family-centered approach. New York: Guilford Press; 2003.

24. Kaminer Y, Burleson JA, Burke R, et al. The efficacy of contingency management for adolescent cannabis use disorder: a controlled study. Subst Abus 2014;35(4):391–8.

25. Ryan SR, Stanger C, Thostenson J, et al. The impact of disruptive behavior disorder on substance use treatment outcome in adolescents. J Subst Abuse Treat 2013;44:506–14.

26. Letourneau EJ, McCart MR, Asuzu K, et al. Caregiver involvement in sexual risk reduction with substance using juvenile delinquents: overview and preliminary outcomes of a randomized trial. Adolesc Psychiatry (Hilversum) 2013;3(4):342–51.

27. McCart MR, Sheidow AJ, Letourneau EJ. Risk reduction therapy for adolescents: targeting substance use and HIV/STI-risk behaviors. Cogn Behav Pract 2014;21(2):161–75.

28. Budney AJ, Marsch LA, Bickel WK. Computerized therapies in the treatment of substance use disorders: toward an addiction treatment technology test. In: el-Guebaly N, Carrà G, Galanter M, editors. Textbook of addiction treatment: international perspectives. Berlin: Springer-Verlag; 2014. p. 987–1006.

Juvenile Drug Treatment Court

David M. Ledgerwood, PhD[a],*, Phillippe B. Cunningham, PhD[b]

KEYWORDS

- Juvenile drug treatment court • Adolescent • Substance use • Cannabis
- Caregivers • Parents • Therapeutic jurisprudence

KEY POINTS

- Juvenile Drug Treatment Courts (JDTCs) were established in the 1990s to reduce the cycle of crime, drug use, and delinquency among youthful offenders.
- JDTCs are made up of multidisciplinary teams, including a judge, district attorneys, public defenders, juvenile probation officers, and drug treatment providers who collaborate to address the unique needs of each participant, guided by the principle of therapeutic jurisprudence.
- The effectiveness of JDTCs has been mixed. Several efforts have been made to improve their effectiveness through further development of the most efficacious components, development of adjunctive treatments designed to improve outcomes, utilization of community resources, and encouragement of family participation.

INTRODUCTION

Substance-abusing and delinquent adolescents involved in the juvenile justice system represent a large and underserved population that is at high risk for significant deleterious outcomes and long-term costs for themselves, their families, their community, and society. Furthermore, without effective interventions, substance-abusing and delinquent adolescents are likely to continue to abuse substances and maintain their criminal activity well into adulthood.[1–3] The costs of substance abuse and crime to society (eg, criminal justice expenditures, fear of crime, pain, and suffering) are staggering, with annual estimates ranging from $820 billion[4] to $3.4 trillion.[5] This article describes Juvenile Drug Treatment Courts (JDTCs), their theoretic underpinnings, common elements and goals, and research-based and practice-informed federal guidelines. The remainder of the article describes how JDTCs operate and summarizes the latest outcome research on their effectiveness.

[a] Department of Psychiatry and Behavioral Neurosciences, Wayne State University, Suite 2A, 3901 Chrysler Drive, Detroit, MI, 48201 USA; [b] Department of Psychiatry and Behavioral Sciences, Division of Global and Community Health, Family Services Research Center, Medical University of South Carolina, 176 Croghan Spur Road, Suite104, Charleston, SC, 29407 USA
* Corresponding author.
E-mail address: dledgerw@med.wayne.edu

Pediatr Clin N Am 66 (2019) 1193–1202
https://doi.org/10.1016/j.pcl.2019.08.011
0031-3955/19/© 2019 Elsevier Inc. All rights reserved.

WHAT ARE JUVENILE DRUG TREATMENT COURTS AND WHAT ARE THEIR COMMON ELEMENTS?

Beginning in the mid-1990s, JDTCs emerged as a promising juvenile justice program model in response to the perceived need to intervene more effectively in reducing the cycle of drug use, crime, and delinquency among youthful offenders. Modeled after the success of adult drug courts in reducing recidivism, a JDTC is a specialized docket within juvenile courts for cases involving youth identified as having problems with alcohol or other drugs severe enough to require treatment. A basic assumption of any JDTC is that youth (and their families) entering court have a complex array of needs that vary considerably from defendant to defendant based on their level of maturation. This assumption is congruent with the theoretic underpinnings of JDTCs, which is the theory of therapeutic jurisprudence (TJ).

TJ asserts that the law and court are social agents for positive therapeutic change.[6] Judicial goals, and the design, operation, procedures, and court personnel (judges, lawyers, probation staff; who value the psychological well-being of its participants), can positively affect criminologic and psychosocial outcomes.[7,8] An essential component of JDTCs, derived from the TJ perspective, is a clear focus on developing treatment and rehabilitative services that can address the unique needs of each youth and his or her family.[7] Consistent with a TJ conceptualization, JDTCs are expected to extend intervention beyond just the youth's substance use and criminal behavior, into his or her mental health (eg, traumatic history, learning disabilities) and that of the family (eg, parental mental health, substance abuse, unemployment, parenting practices, practical needs). That is, from the TJ lens, JDTCs are family focused and expected to play an important role in connecting youth and their families with services needed to address the myriad social and practical factors (eg, poor parenting practices, inadequate housing, limited employment and vocational activities, lack of social support) that contribute directly or indirectly to a youth's substance use and criminal offending.

Although JDTCs may differ across jurisdictions, they all share several common therapeutic elements and goals. At their core, JDTCs provide substance-abusing youth offenders with specialized treatment and rehabilitative services that require effective partnering with a youth's family to address substance use and prevent legal problems.[8] To establish effective relationships with families requires JDTCs to maintain a creative problem-solving stance built on the principles of collaboration, case management, and a balance between treatment and accountability,[9] with a clear focus to maximize therapeutic benefits while recognizing and maintaining legal safeguards (due process, community safety).[10,11] Other common therapeutic elements of JDTCs include immediate intervention and continuous supervision of the youth/family (parent or guardian); treatment and rehabilitative services to address the unique needs of each youth/family; judicial oversight and coordination of services (treatment, education, social services) to promote accountability across systems (youth, family, treatment providers, probation staff, and so forth); and immediate judicial response to youth/family noncompliance with treatment or court requirements.[7]

These common elements have been codified by leading drug treatment court organizations (National Drug Court Institute, a division of the National Association of Drug Court Professionals, and the National Council of Juvenile and Family Court Judges) into 5 goals for JDTC programs. As suggested by these organizations, the goals of any JDTC are to (1) provide immediate intervention and treatment of offenders through ongoing oversight and monitoring by the court; (2) improve an offender's psychosocial functioning across each domain of functional impairments (eg, social, familial, academic) contributing to their drug use or criminal offending; (3) provide offenders with the necessary skills to lead productive lives free of substances and crime; (4) help strengthen the offender's family functioning to improve their capacity to provide the necessary structure to effectively monitor and guide their child; and (5) promote accountability by all involved systems (eg, family, school, probation, treatment, and rehabilitative service providers).[12]

JUVENILE DRUG TREATMENT COURT GUIDELINES

Between December 2003 and June 2013, the number of JDTCs increased from 268 to 476 courts. In June 2015, there were an estimated 409 JDCs operating in the United States.[13] As JDTCs proliferated, mixed evidence of their effectiveness began to emerge in the scientific literature. In the mid-2000s, several reviews and meta-analyses reported only modest effect sizes and slight reductions in recidivism among program participants.[14–17] In response to these mixed findings and to increase the effectiveness of JDTCs, the Office of Juvenile Justice and Delinquency Prevention (OJJDP), in partnership with the scientific community, conducted a systematic review of the extant literature. The goal was to synthesize the available evidence from JDTCs to identify implementation components associated with the most positive outcomes to create research-based and practice-informed guidelines for JDTCs.[18] This review also included research from the fields of drug treatment, juvenile justice, and effective interventions in child welfare, public health, and education. This effort resulted in OJJDP publishing Juvenile Drug Treatment Court Guidelines (**Table 1**), which can be found at https://www.ojjdp.gov/Juvenile-Drug-Treatment-Court-Guidelines.html.

Ultimately, the focus of these guidelines is to ensure improved JDTC outcomes by making sure these courts promote adolescent development, reduce substance use, and reduce delinquency.[19] Concerning healthy adolescent development, implicit in these guidelines is a realization that courts must inculcate a developmental perspective that understands the importance of improving family functioning, personal well-being, healthy family and peer relationships, and educational/vocational functioning.[19]

According to the federal eligibility guidelines, JDTCs should only serve those youth who meet eligibility criteria. These eligibility criteria include the following: youth with a substance use disorder based on assessments from validated risk and needs

Table 1 OJJDP juvenile treatment court guidelines	
Objectives	**Guideline**
1	Focus the JDTC philosophy and practice on effectively addressing substance use and criminogenic needs to decrease future offending and substance use and to increase positive outcomes
2	Ensure equitable treatment of all youth by adhering to eligibility criteria and conducting an initial screening
3	Provide a JDTC process that engages the full team and follows procedures fairly
4	Conduct comprehensive needs assessments that inform individualized case management
5	Implement contingency management, case management, and community supervision strategies effectively
6	Refer participants to evidence-based substance use treatment, to other services, and for prosocial connections
7	Monitor and track program completion and termination

instruments (eg, urinalysis, global appraisal of individual needs); youth aged 14 to 17.5 years; and youth with moderate to high risk of reoffending (eg, nonviolent, first-time offenders). In most jurisdictions, youth adjudicated for a violent or sexual-oriented offense are ineligible for a JDTC.

HOW DO JUVENILE DRUG TREATMENT COURTS OPERATE?

JDTCs take a multidisciplinary team approach in addressing the unique needs of each participant. A multidisciplinary team of professionals, who take a nonadversarial team approach, coordinate the day-to-day operations of the court and provide a wide range of complementary services germane to healthy child development and public safety. JDTC teams include a judge, court coordinator/supervisor, district or prosecuting attorney, defense attorney or public defender, case manager or probation officer, and a substance abuse treatment provider (roles of each member of the JDTC team are summarized in **Table 2**). Teams may also include a school representative, as well as representatives from child welfare, social services, and adult counseling services (eg, parents who may require their own mental health services or educational/vocational counseling). Each member of the team reviews a participant's progress since the last status hearing and makes legal or treatment recommendations based on the results of their respective assessments. The latter occurs during weekly team meetings designed to provide the judge with information to inform their decision during the upcoming status hearing.

JDTC status hearings (legal proceedings) typically occur every 1 to 4 weeks where the judge has an opportunity to review each participant's progress (eg, treatment, school, home, community). During the hearing, a participant is called before the judge with his or her caregiver and accompanied by their defense attorney or public defender. The judge may ask the adolescent participant to give an update on how well (or not) the youth has been doing since the last hearing. Caregivers are also asked to provide their own independent evaluation of the youth's progress. The judge then directs members of the team to provide their assessment of the youth's progress, and results from the most recent urine drug screen (UDS). Once the review is complete, the judge makes a decision to provide an incentive (ie, reward) for compliance or sanction for noncompliance (ie, not meeting program requirements).[20]

Consistent with operant learning principles, the judge selects from a wide range of available incentives for program compliance (eg, abstinence, school/treatment attendance) and sanctions for noncompliance (eg, positive UDS, failure to attend treatment, truancy), to help youth progress through program phases (see later discussion). Successful progression through each phase (individual courts may have 3 to 5 phases) can last anywhere from 6 to 12 months. Phase progression is facilitated by immediate and contingent consequences designed to reinforce or modify the behavior of the participant and his or her family.[21] Incentives for program compliance may include praise and encouragement from the judge, gifts (eg, movie passes, tokens, gift cards, tickets to sporting events), less frequent court appearances or UDSs, and ultimately, graduation. Sanctions for noncompliance or noncompliant events (eg, drug relapse, law violations, unexcused absence from treatment, court, or school, inappropriate dress, inappropriate behavior in court) may range from a verbal warning to brief detention (hours to days/weekends) in a juvenile facility. Sanctions may also include community service or a writing assignment. A major law violation (eg, felony) often results in immediate termination from JDTC.

Each phase has a specific focus and requirements designed to hold participants accountable and to track their progress in areas pertinent to adolescent development,

Table 2
Roles and responsibilities of juvenile drug treatment court team members

Team Member	Roles and Responsibilities
Judge	• Presides over court proceedings and makes all final decisions regarding a youth participant's involvement, including treatment, incentives, and sanctions • Reviews weekly status reports for each adolescent (usually during a team meeting where members provide updates on each participant), which detail their compliance with treatment and the treatment provider, drug testing, progress at home and school, and progress toward abstinence and obeying the law. • Administers a system of graduated sanctions and rewards during hearings to increase each participant's accountability and to enhance the likelihood of abstinence
District attorney	• Takes a nonadversarial stance and balances role of prosecutor (ie, maintaining public safety) with the rehabilitative needs of the participant • Collaborates with the treatment team in monitoring the youth's progress, and makes recommendations regarding sanctions and treatment recommendations • Attends weekly status and other court hearings (eg, detention, probation violations, revocations, and any other special hearings associated with a JDTC participant) • Reviews weekly progress reports of each case, and if a youth is rearrested, reviews each new charge and assesses the appropriateness of the youth's continued participation in JDTC
Public defender	• Attorney who works for a public offender's office, which is a government-funded agency that represents indigent criminal defendants • Responsible for ensuring participant's legal and constitutional rights are not violated in court proceedings • Promotes participant health and well-being • Attends weekly status hearings, appears at all court hearings and proceedings, reviews weekly progress reports, and takes a nonadversarial stance with the court • Negotiates legal and treatment recommendations consistent with participant needs
Juvenile probation officer	• Assigned to JDTCs by the Department of Probation and provides quality assurance for each youth's participation in the program • Responsible for the direct supervision of each participant's compliance with court mandates (eg, sanctions, recommendations) • Oversees implementation of an appropriate level of supervision in the community, serving as a liaison with relevant agencies (eg, Department of Health and Human Services, adolescent treatment providers, school), and monitoring the day-to-day activities and home environment of each participant
Drug treatment provider	• Participates in the weekly status hearings • Makes treatment recommendations to the court based on the specific needs of each youth and family (eg, mental health, social services, and so forth) and provides weekly updates as needed • Provides the multidisciplinary team with information regarding the adolescent's attendance and participation in treatment (substance abuse, mental health) • Levels of care available to JDTC usually include outpatient treatment, intensive outpatient treatment, hospital-based detoxification, and short-term (30-day) and long-term (60–90 day) residential treatment

relapse prevention, and aftercare. The team tracks and reviews drug abstinence (results from the most recent UDS), school attendance, grades, and behavior at home (eg, compliance with caregiver behavioral expectations, curfew compliance). In phase 1, the focus is often on participant stabilization with the following requirements: weekly status hearing (ie, drug court attendance), drug treatment and random UDS, regular school attendance, weekly contact with the assigned juvenile probation officer, and obeying the law. With a continued focus on school and treatment attendance, phase 2 adds a primary focus on drug abstinence, and begins aftercare planning. In the final phase 3, the primary focus is transitioning to aftercare and JDTC graduation. A major benefit for graduation from a JDTC, in addition to reducing or eliminating drug use, is that an offender's criminal record is sealed or expunged by the court.

CHARACTERISTICS OF THOSE WHO PARTICIPATE

Youth who participate in JDTCs vary based on the demographics and policies of the various jurisdictions, but there are some commonalities. Several studies have found that male youth make up more than 80% of JDTC enrollees.[22-27] Racial and ethnic minorities are also overrepresented among JDTCs. For example, an early investigation in the Orange County JDTC revealed that just over half of the youth were white and 35% were African American.[28] In a large clinical trial by Henggeler and colleagues,[23] conducted in a JDTC in South Carolina, 67% of youth were African American, 31% were white, and 2% were biracial. Similarly, a study conducted in Birmingham, Alabama, recruited 71% African American youth.[27] Dakof and colleagues[22] also found high proportions of African American (33%–39%) and Hispanic (56%–62%) youth in their clinical trial conducted in Miami-Dade Florida.

Families of JDTC participants are often characterized by single parenthood and poverty. Henggeler and colleagues[23] found that 52% of JDTC youth lived with a single biological or adoptive parent, and only 21% lived with both biological parents. Furthermore, primary caregivers had a median 12th grade education and a median family income ranging from US$10,000 to US$15,000, with 38% of families receiving public assistance. Similarly, Henggeler and colleagues[24] found that 53% lived with a single biological parent, median household income ranged from US$$20,000 to US$30,000, and 47% were receiving assistance. Sloan and colleagues[27] reported that about 67% of JDTC participants lived in a single-parent home. Dakof and colleagues[22] found that more than 50% of participants lived in a single-parent home, with a median family income around US$20,000 or less. Other studies have found similar rates of single-parent households and low family income.[25] Liddle and colleagues[25] also found that 75% of teens had a parent with criminal justice system involvement.

Cannabis use was the most frequently used illicit substance across JDTC studies, with rates as high as 98%.[22-25,28] These studies also showed alcohol abuse and dependence to be prevalent, whereas use of other substances (eg, cocaine, opioids) was relatively uncommon. In many cases, drug-related offenses were the most common crimes that resulted in JDTC referral.[27,28]

Psychiatric comorbidity is prevalent among youth attending JDTCs. High rates of externalizing disorders (eg, conduct disorder, oppositional defiant disorder, attention deficit disorder) have been reported in several studies.[22-24] These studies also found increased rates of internalizing disorders (eg, anxiety disorders, major depression, obsessive-compulsive disorder).

Overall, JDTC studies reveal that most teens experience several disadvantages. Many identify as African American or Hispanic and come from socioeconomically disadvantaged homes often headed by a single caregiver. Most use marijuana, but other drugs of abuse are also present. Finally, many experience significant internalizing and externalizing psychiatric disorders that have the potential to interfere with the drug court process.

DRUG COURT EFFECTIVENESS

Recent research examining the effectiveness of JDTCs has provided mixed results. One meta-analysis of 46 evaluation studies, for example, revealed that JDTCs were no more or less effective than usual court proceedings.[29] However, the investigators noted a great deal of variability in study findings and criticized the research literature as using mostly poor methodology and lacking randomized trials. Another meta-analysis found that JDTCs had a modest positive effect on recidivism, but that the effects tended to be less pronounced among the more rigorous clinical trials.[27]

Individually, several studies have provided evidence for the effectiveness of JDTCs. In one of the most rigorous studies to date, Henggeler and colleagues[23] revealed that JDTCs resulted in decreased alcohol and polysubstance use and fewer criminal offenses during the follow-up period compared with family court. In another study, a retrospective examination comparing 24-month post-drug court reincarceration rates found that JDTC was comparable with a more intensive intervention that incorporated continuation of pre-adjudicatory probation, dropping charges on program completion, drug education and treatment, parenting classes, and urinalysis monitoring.[27]

Cost-effectiveness analyses have shown JDTCs to have some advantages over family courts. For example, Sheidow and colleagues[30] found that although JDTC was more than 3 times the cost of family court, it was still more cost-effective for reducing criminal behavior. Cost-effectiveness was similar between the 2 court types for substance abuse outcomes.

Other studies have revealed specific youth characteristics that may predict success in JDTC. For example, a secondary analysis of data from Henggeler and colleagues[23] examined youth-based (pre-treatment marijuana use, arrests, anxiety/depression), family-level (caregiver illegal substance use, family legal problems, parental supervision), and extrafamilial (peer drug activities, school status, treatment condition) variables.[31] Only 1 variable, parental illegal substance use, predicted treatment nonresponse as measured by continued cannabis use. Thus, it may be important to consider and encourage treatment of caregiver substance use problems for teens who are engaged in JDTCs.

Community collaboration is viewed as an essential way to improve drug court services. In a qualitative study of drug court representatives, Korchmaros and colleagues[32] found that community collaboration, engaging families, and improved service matching are key features that would enhance JDTC effectiveness. However, there are barriers in each of these areas. For example, engaging families in their teens' JDTC process is difficult in part because families may be unable or unwilling to participate. Thus, strategies to reduce such barriers are viewed as essential for improving effectiveness.

EFFORTS TO IMPROVE DRUG COURT USING EVIDENCE-BASED TREATMENTS

Given the mixed findings to date with regard to JDTC, there has been an effort to improve outcomes by incorporating evidence-based treatment (EBT) and conducting clinical trials to examine whether these adjunctive therapies might improve primarily substance use or criminal recidivism outcomes. To date, most of the studies that have explored the use of EBTs have used individual behavioral interventions such as contingency management (CM) treatment, or family-based interventions such as multisystemic therapy (MST).[33]

Henggeler and colleagues[23] conducted a randomized clinical trial to examine the relative efficacy of 4 treatment conditions: (1) family court; (2) JDTC alone; (3) JDTC plus MST; or (4) MST plus a CM intervention where teens could receive reinforcement for target behaviors related to drug abstinence (MST + CM). As already noted, participants who received JDTC had better outcomes than did those who attended family court. This study also found that teens randomly assigned to MST and MST + CM conditions experienced significantly greater drug abstinence than those assigned to JDTC alone, as measured by UDS. JDTC conditions demonstrated improvements in recidivism measures relative to family court, but addition of MST or CM did not improve rates further. Results of this study showed that the addition of an EBT (in this case MST and CM) significantly improved the cost-effectiveness of JDTC.[30]

In a second trial by this group, Henggeler and colleagues[24] randomly assigned 6 JDTCs to provide a treatment that included either family engagement and contingency management interventions (CM-FAM) or to continue to provide treatment as usual. In total, 104 juvenile offenders received treatment over an 18-month period. Participants in the CM-FAM condition exhibited significant reductions in marijuana use as measured by UDS data (but not self-report) compared with treatment as usual. CM-FAM participants also experienced significantly greater decreases in general delinquency, offenses against persons, and property offenses compared with usual care.

Another clinical trial by Dakof and colleagues[22] randomized JDTC participants to an EBT, multidimensional family therapy, or adolescent group therapy (which is somewhat more consistent with treatments typically provided in JDTC). Both groups experienced significantly reduced offending and substance abuse at 6-month follow-up, and improvements in self-reported delinquency at 24 months. Over the longer term, substance use and re-arrest rates tended to worsen, but did not reach baseline levels. Multidimensional family therapy was associated with fewer felony arrests and less substance use at 24-month follow-up compared with adolescent group therapy. Clearly, adding evidence-based family therapy resulted in significantly better long-term outcomes than a more traditional treatment approach.

Taken together, these studies demonstrate that the addition of EBTs to JDTC may enhance the efficacy of these interventions. However, relatively few studies have tested the incorporation of EBTs into the JDTC model.

SUMMARY

JDTCs are one of the few promising juvenile justice interventions that help substance-abusing offenders turn their lives around by providing specialized treatment services and intensive judicial supervision as an alternative to incarceration. Overall, JDTCs provide an opportunity for justice-involved youth to receive help for substance abuse and mental health problems rather than confinement in juvenile detention. However, the results of research conducted thus far have demonstrated that JDTCs are not universally effective at reducing recidivism and substance use. Further, there are relatively few trials designed to test adjunctive treatment to JDTCs, but those that have been conducted demonstrate that addition EBTs can be used to bolster their effectiveness. Recommended future directions include assessment of factors that affect JDTC effectiveness and development and testing of adjunct treatments that may help to engage families into the JDTC process.

ACKNOWLEDGMENTS

This work was supported by National Institutes of Health Grant R01MD011322 awarded to co-principal investigators: P.B.C. and D.M.L.

REFERENCES

1. Godley SH, Godley MD, Dennis ML. The assertive aftercare protocol for adolescent substance abusers. In: Wagner EF, Waldron HB, editors. Innovations in adolescent substance abuse interventions. New York: Pergamon; 2001. p. 313–31.
2. Henggeler SW, Clingempeel WG, Brondino MJ, et al. Four- year follow-up of multisystemic therapy with substance abusing and dependent juvenile offenders. J Am Acad Child Adolesc Psychiatry 2002;41:868–74.
3. Liberman AM, editor. The long view of crime: a synthesis of longitudinal research. New York: Springer; 2008.
4. National Institute on Drug Abuse. Trends and statistics 2018. Available at: https://www.drugabuse.gov/related-topics/trends-statistics. Accessed January 9, 2019.
5. Government Accountability Office. Costs of crime: experts report challenges estimating costs and suggests improvements to better inform policy decisions. GAO publication no. 17-732. Washington, DC.: U.S. Government Printing Office; 2017.
6. Wexler D. Therapeutic jurisprudence: an overview. Disability law symposium issue: legal and treatment issues. Thomas M Cooley L Rev 2000;17:125–34.
7. Gilbert J, Grimm R, Parnham J. Applying therapeutic prinicples to a family-focused juvenile justice model (delinquency). Ala Law Rev 2001;52:1153.
8. Shaffer DK. Looking inside the black box of drug courts: a meta-analytic review. Justice Q 2011;28:493–521.
9. van Wormer J, Lutze F. Exploring the evidence: the value of juvenile drug courts." Juvenile and family justice today 2011. Available at: http://www.ncjfcj.org/sites/default/files/jdc%20evidence.pdf. Accessed April 6, 2019.
10. Rottman D, Casey P. Therapeutic jurisprudence and the emergence of problem-solving courts. Rockville (MD): National Institute of Justice Journal; 1999. p. 12–9.
11. Winick BJ. Therapeutic jurisprudence and problem solving courts. Fordham Urban Law J 2003;30:1055–103.
12. National Association of Drug Court Professionals. Defining drug courts: the key components. Alexandria (VA): National Association of Drug Court Professionals; 2004. Available at: https://www.ncjrs.gov/pdffiles1/bja/205621.pdf. Accessed May 10, 2019.
13. National Criminal Justice Reference System. In the spotlight: Drug courts - facts and figures. Available at: https://www.ncjrs.gov/spotlight/drug_courts/facts.html. Accessed September 17, 2019.
14. Aos S, Miller M, Drake E. Evidence-based public policy options to reduce future prison construction, criminal justice costs, and crime rates. Olympia (WA): Washington State Institute for Public Policy; 2006.
15. Latimer J, Morton-Bourgon K, Chretien J. A meta-analytic examination of drug treatment courts: do they reduce recidivism? Ottawa (Ontario): Department of Justice Canada; 2006.
16. Shafer DK. Reconsidering drug court effectiveness: a meta-analytic review. Diss Abstr Int 2006;67:09A (AAT No. 323113).
17. Wilson DB, Mitchell O, MacKenzie DL. A systematic review of drug court effects on recidivism. J Exp Criminol 2006;2:459–87.
18. Wilson D, Olaghere A, Kimbrell CS. Developing juvenile drug court practices on process standards: a systematic review and qualitative synthesis. Washington

(DC): Office of Juvenile Justice and Delinquency Prevention, Office of Justice Programs, U.S. Department of Justice; 2016.

19. Office of Juvenile Justice Delinquency Prevention. Juvenile drug treatment court guidelines. Washington, DC: U.S. Department of Justice, Office of Justice Programs; 2016.

20. Festinger DS, Marlowe DB, Lee PA, et al. Status hearings in drug court: when more is less and less is more. Drug Alcohol Depend 2002;2:151–7.

21. Gatowski S, Miller NB, Rubin SM, et al. OJJDP juvenile drug treatment court guidelines project: juvenile drug treatment court listening sessions. Washington, DC: U.S. Department of Justice; 2016.

22. Dakof GA, Henderson CE, Rowe CL, et al. A randomized clinical trial of family therapy in juvenile drug court. J Fam Psychol 2015;29:232–41.

23. Henggeler SW, Halliday-Boykins CA, Cunningham PB, et al. Juvenile drug court: enhancing outcomes by integrating evidence-based treatments. J Consult Clin Psychol 2006;74:42–54.

24. Henggeler SW, McCart M, Cunningham PB, et al. Enhancing the effectiveness of juvenile drug courts by integrating evidence-based practices. J Consult Clin Psychol 2012;80:264–75.

25. Liddle HA, Dakof GA, Henderson C, et al. Implementation outcomes of multidimensional family therapy-detention to community: a reintegration program for drug-using juvenile detainees. Int J Offender Ther Comp Criminol 2011;55:587–604.

26. Mitchel O, Wilson DB, Eggers A, et al. Assessing the effectiveness of drug courts on recidivism: a meta-analytic review of traditional and non-traditional drug courts. J Crim Justice 2012;40:60–71.

27. Sloan JJ, Smykla JO, Rush JP. Do juvenile drug courts reduce recidivism?: outcomes of drug court and an adolescent substance abuse program. Am J Crim Justice 2004;29:95–115.

28. Applegate BK, Santana S. Intervening with youthful substance abusers: a preliminary analysis of juvenile drug court. Justice System Journal 2000;21:281–300.

29. Tanner-Smith EE, Lipsey MW, Wilson DB. Juvenile drug court effects on recidivism and drug use: a systematic review and meta-analysis. J Exp Criminol 2016;12:477–513.

30. Sheidow AJ, Jayawardhana J, Bradford D, et al. Money matters: cost-effectiveness of juvenile drug court with and without evidence-based treatments. J Child Adolesc Subst Abuse 2012;21:69–90.

31. Halliday-Boykins CA, Schaeffer CM, Henggeler SW, et al. Predicting nonresponse to juvenile drug court interventions. J Subst Abuse Treat 2010;39:318–28.

32. Korchmaros JD, Thompson-Dyck K, Haring RC. Professionals' perceptions of and recommendations for matching juvenile drug court clients to services. Child Youth Serv Rev 2017;73:149–64.

33. Henggeler SW, Schoenwald SK, Borduin CM, et al. Multisystemic therapy for antisocial behavior in children and adolescents. 2nd edition. New York: Guilford Press; 2009.

Technology-Delivered Interventions for Substance Use Among Adolescents

Steven J. Ondersma, PhD[a],*, Jennifer D. Ellis, MA[b],
Stella M. Resko, PhD[c], Emily Grekin, PhD[d]

KEYWORDS

- Adolescence • Technology • Substance use • Interventions • Brief interventions
- Review

KEY POINTS

- Technology-delivered interventions for adolescents with unhealthy substance use may help to address significant challenges regarding reach, fidelity, and cost.
- At present, most work in this area involves either brief interventions in school or health care settings, or multisession preventive interventions for school or community settings.
- Early findings provide mixed support for technology-delivered interventions for alcohol and/or drug use among adolescents.
- Much of the current literature in this area has a range of methodological limitations that weaken confidence in findings.
- Future trials in this area should consistently adhere to best practices, including preregistration, controlling for alpha inflation, large sample sizes, collection of biomarker data, best practices to ensure high follow-up rates, and using imputation for missing outcome data.

Nearly half of adolescents report lifetime use of an illicit drug, most commonly marijuana, and 14% of 12th graders report having had 5 or more alcoholic drinks at

Disclosure: Dr S.J. Ondersma discloses part ownership of a company marketing e-intervention authoring software to investigators and health care providers. Dr. Ondersma's effort on this review was supported by Helene Lycacki/Joe Young Sr. funds from the State of Michigan. The other authors have no disclosures to report.
[a] Department of Psychiatry and Behavioral Neurosciences, Merrill Palmer Skillman Institute, Wayne State University, 71 East Ferry Avenue, Detroit, MI 48202, USA; [b] Department of Psychology, Wayne Statue University, 5057 Woodward Avenue, Detroit, MI 48202, USA; [c] School of Social Work and Merrill Palmer Skillman Institute, Wayne State University, 5447 Woodward Avenue, Detroit, MI 48202, USA; [d] Department of Psychology, Wayne State University, 5057 Woodward Avenue, Detroit, MI 48202, USA
* Corresponding author.
E-mail address: s.ondersma@wayne.edu
Twitter: @steveondersma (S.J.O.)

a time in the past 2 weeks.[1] Substance use during adolescence is associated with a wide range of short-term and long-term negative outcomes. Adolescents reporting use of alcohol, marijuana, or other substances are at increased risk of violence exposure,[2] academic failure,[3–5] delinquency,[6,7] and suicide.[8–10] Further, still-developing neural pathways can be negatively and persistently affected by introduction of substance use during this critical period,[11] a phenomenon that may partly explain the increased likelihood of drug use in adulthood for adolescents who use marijuana before age 17 years.[12,13]

Research has identified a range of evidence-based treatments for unhealthy substance use among adolescents.[14] However, these evidence-based interventions, as with those for adults, reach only a small proportion of those who could benefit from treatment,[15] and are difficult to disseminate with fidelity to the original model.[16,17] These challenges have led to calls for broader approaches with impact on a population level rather than only on the treatment-seeking minority.[18,19]

Technology may help address challenges related to reach and fidelity. As has often been noted, technology-delivered interventions can be accessed at any time and from any place and can be delivered far more cheaply than person-delivered treatments, thus helping to address health disparities. In addition, technology-delivered interventions do not require widespread training or supervision to implement, do not require retraining when updated, and are not limited by geography, enabling access in rural areas. Technology-delivered interventions also facilitate fine-grained research into specific elements that drive or hinder positive effects. Recognition of these advantages has led to a rapidly growing literature evaluating technology-delivered interventions specifically for adolescents and young adults.

This article reviews that literature in 4 specific subgroups: brief interventions, text-messaging interventions, interventions leveraging social media, and multisession interventions. Note that there are many more technology-delivered interventions available than are reported in this article; attention here is restricted to those for which evaluation data regarding substance use outcomes have been published in a peer-reviewed journal. This article also restricts its focus to interventions that have been designed and evaluated in controlled studies (either randomized or with a comparison group) for use with adolescents less than 18 years of age.

BRIEF MOTIVATIONAL INTERVENTIONS
Brief Interventions with At-Risk Samples

Computer-delivered and Web-based interventions for substance use are common among both college students[20] and non–college-attending adults.[21] However, few studies have tested these interventions among adolescents. Existing studies in this area have evaluated interventions with adolescents in health care settings, such as emergency department and primary care,[22–25] as well as with school-based and community samples.[26–28]

Results from studies conducted in health care settings have yielded mixed results. Walton and colleagues[25] recruited 328 adolescents who reported past-year cannabis use from urban community health clinics. All participants were randomized to a computer-delivered brief intervention (CBI), a therapist-delivered brief intervention (TBI), or a control condition (ie, informational brochure). Both interventions were motivational interviewing (MI) based and included tailored feedback, decisional balance exercises, goal setting, and skills training for difficult situations. Participants in all 3 groups completed online follow-up assessments of cannabis use, cannabis consequences, driving under the influence of cannabis, alcohol use, and other drug use at 3, 6, and 12 months postbaseline. Notably, neither intervention significantly reduced cannabis use over the course of the study. However, the CBI reduced cannabis consequences (at 3-month follow-up) as well as other drug use (at 3-month and 6-month follow-up), whereas the TBI reduced driving under the influence of cannabis (6-month follow-up).

Cunningham and colleagues[23] recruited 836 adolescents with a positive screen on the Alcohol Use Disorders Identification Test–Consumption (AUDIT-C; the first 3 items of the full 10-item AUDIT)[29] from an urban emergency department. As in Walton and colleagues[25] (2013), participants were randomized to a CBI, a TBI, or a control condition (an informational brochure). The tailored interventions were MI based, and the CBI was set up as a Facebook-style program in which participants chose virtual friends to interact with throughout the intervention. Participants in all 3 groups completed self-report measures of alcohol use, alcohol consequences, driving under the influence of alcohol, alcohol-related injury, and drug use at 3 and 12 months postbaseline. In addition, some participants received a booster session of TBI at the 6-month follow-up. Both the CBI and the TBI reduced alcohol consumption (3-month follow-up), alcohol consequences (3-month and 12-month follow-up), and prescription drug use (12-month follow-up). CBI also reduced driving under the influence, whereas the TBI reduced alcohol-related injury (12-month follow-up). The booster session reduced alcohol consequences, but only for those who were in the control condition at baseline.

Walton and colleagues[24] recruited 726 adolescents who reported both past-year alcohol use and aggression from an urban emergency department. All participants

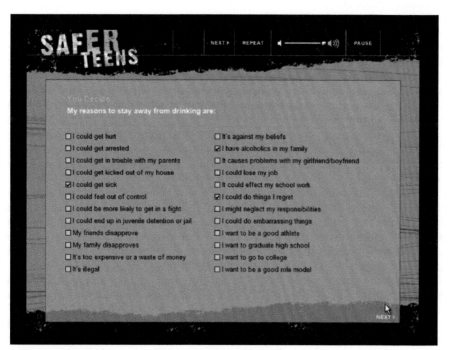

Fig. 1. Safer Teens program. (Image courtesy of Maureen Walton, PhD, and Rebecca Cunningham, MD, 2012.)

were randomized to a CBI (the Safer Teens intervention; **Fig. 1**), a TBI, or a control condition (an informational brochure). As in the previous studies, the interventions (which targeted both alcohol use and violence) were MI based and used techniques such as feedback, decisional balance, and skills training. Follow-up surveys assessing alcohol use, binge drinking, alcohol consequences, violence, and violence consequences were administered at 3 and 6 months postbaseline. Compared with participants in the control group, those in the CBI group reported reductions in alcohol consequences (6-month follow-up). Participants in the TBI group reported reductions in peer aggression, peer violence, and violence consequences at the 3-month follow-up, and reported reductions in alcohol consequences at the 6-month follow-up. Notably, there were no significant reductions in alcohol use for CBI or TBI. In a 12-month follow-up study using the same sample, Cunningham and colleagues[22] reported that although participants in the TBI group showed reductions in peer aggression and victimization, neither intervention was associated with improvements in alcohol-related outcomes.

Computer-based intervention trials recruiting adolescents from community or school-based settings have also yielded mixed results. For example, Voogt and colleagues[28] recruited 609 heavy-drinking students from vocational schools in the Netherlands. Participants were cluster randomized by school to either an online alcohol intervention (the What Do You Drink program, an MI-based intervention that includes normed feedback, goal setting, education, and drinking refusal skill practice) or a control condition (no intervention). Weekly alcohol consumption, heavy drinking, and binge drinking were assessed at 1-month and 6-month follow-up. Results revealed no intervention effects on any alcohol outcomes at either follow-up. Notably, this study had large attrition rates of 35.5% and 54% at 1-month and 6-month follow-up, respectively.

Arnaud and colleagues[26] recruited a convenience sample of 1449 adolescents to complete a fully automated, Web-based brief motivational intervention (the WISEteens intervention). Participants were recruited through leaflets, flyers, and online advertisements. Adolescents who screened positive for at-risk alcohol or other drug use (using the CRAFFT) were randomized to either the WISEteens intervention or an assessment-only control condition. Past-month alcohol use, binge drinking, illegal drug use, and polydrug use were assessed at a 3-month follow-up. Because only 14.5% of the sample provided follow-up data, investigators used expectation maximization imputation for outcome analyses. Results suggested that the intervention group had greater reductions in past-month alcohol use than the control group, as well as greater reduction in drinking quantity. There were no intervention effects on drug use.

McCarty and colleagues[27] recruited 148 adolescents meeting criteria for moderate-risk to high-risk alcohol use from urban, school-based health centers. During their health center visit, participants were randomized to either complete or not complete an online program that provided tailored, motivational feedback about substance use (the Check Yourself tool). At 2-month follow-up, participants in the intervention group reported that they had received more substance use counseling from their provider during their health center visit. They also reported greater motivation to reduce marijuana use. However, there were no group differences in any alcohol or marijuana use outcomes.

Knight and colleagues[30] examined the use of a computer-facilitated screening and brief intervention (CSBI) program in which adolescents in a pediatric health care setting received computer-facilitated screening, feedback, and psychoeducation regarding substance use, and their health care providers had access to the screening results and talking points. In a sample of 211 adolescents reporting alcohol or drug use in the previous 12 months, Knight and colleagues[30] found that the CSBI was associated with significantly longer time to first postbaseline marijuana use but not time to first alcohol use or heavy episodic alcohol use.

Brief Interventions with Universal Samples

Technology-delivered brief interventions have also been used with universal/unselected samples (thus seeking to prevent the onset of substance use and/or to reduce substance use that is already present). Three trials by Doumas and colleagues[31–33] tested eCHECKUP TO GO, a 30-minute, Web-delivered, feedback-based intervention originally designed for drinking among college students,[34] for its ability to prevent alcohol use and related consequences among high school students. Technology-delivered personalized normed feedback interventions typically ask questions regarding frequency of use, experience of consequences, money and time spent on alcohol, and so forth, and then show images providing feedback regarding how their frequency of use and related consequences compare with those of their peers. In the 2014 article, using a sample of 513 ninth grade students from one of 2 junior high schools (with 1 randomly designated as the intervention school and 1 the control school), Doumas and colleagues[31] found positive intervention-related effects for 4 of 7 outcomes, including drinking frequency, at a 3-month follow-up.

In the second trial from this group,[32] 221 high school seniors were randomly assigned to either the eCHECKUP TO GO intervention or to a control condition. Receipt of the intervention was associated with positive effects on 2 of 4 outcomes (weekly drinking quantity and peak drinking quantity) at a 6-week follow-up. The third trial[33] randomly assigned 105 high school seniors to the eCHECKUP TO GO intervention or to control, and found no between-group effects on alcohol-related consequences at a 30-day follow-up, but did find significant group differences on alcohol-related consequences at a 6-month follow-up.

Knight and colleagues[35] also tested a brief eHealth intervention for substance use among adolescents. As described earlier, their intervention was introduced to youth during routine health care encounters, and leveraged that setting by also incorporating input from health care providers. Harris and colleagues[36] tested this intervention approach in a sample of 2685 adolescents aged 12 to 18 years, recruited from 9 clinics in New England and 10 in Prague, Czech Republic. Adolescents whose health care encounters took place following intervention implementation showed less alcohol use at 3-month and 12-month follow-ups (US sample only) as well as less marijuana use at 3 and 12 months (Prague sample only) than adolescents who were seen before intervention implementation. Later reanalysis showed significant reductions in heavy episodic drinking in the Prague sample at the 3-month follow-up, but not at the 12-month follow-up, and no changes at any time point in the New England sample.

TEXT-MESSAGING INTERVENTIONS

Data from the Pew Research Center suggest that, as of 2018, 95% of adolescents, across gender, racial and ethnic groups, and socioeconomic status, have access to a smartphone,[37] and texting remains the most common way that adolescents communicate with one another.[38] Given the high levels of access to and use of smartphones among adolescents, text message–delivered interventions represent a promising platform for intervention delivery. However, few studies to date have examined the efficacy of text message–delivered interventions in reducing alcohol or drug use among adolescents.

Text-Messaging Interventions for Identified Risk

The authors were unable to identify any controlled trials of text messaging–based interventions focused exclusively on either alcohol or drug use among adolescents less than 18 years of age. However, Haug and colleagues[39] recruited tobacco users and randomized participants to either a tobacco-focused intervention or a combined tobacco and alcohol intervention.[39] Using a sample of secondary school students who reported smoking at least 4 cigarettes in the previous month and 1 cigarette in the previous week, Haug and colleagues[39] randomized participants into either a 3-month text-messaging intervention designed to reduce tobacco smoking or a 3-month text-messaging intervention with Web-based normed feedback designed to reduce both tobacco and alcohol consumption. Although there were no overall group differences on smoking, the combined smoking/alcohol intervention was more effective than the smoking-only intervention at reducing 7-day smoking abstinence among those reporting higher levels of alcohol consumption. This finding suggests that consideration of other substance use may be important in tailoring text message–delivered interventions.

Text-Messaging Interventions with Universal Samples

Text messaging can also be used to prevent substance use initiation and/or reduce current use among unselected samples (such as with entire classrooms). For example, Haug and colleagues[40] randomly assigned 1355 students (mean age, 16.8 years) to either a Web-based brief intervention followed by a text-messaging intervention that was tailored to level of risk, or a control condition. Participants in the intervention condition reported significantly less binge drinking in the past 30 days (defined as 5 or more standard drinks on a single occasion for boys, and 4 or more for girls) at the single 6-month follow-up. Effects were not seen on binge frequency, quantity of alcohol, or peak blood alcohol concentration.

INTERVENTIONS THROUGH SOCIAL MEDIA

Given the widespread usage of social media among adolescents,[37] social media presents a particularly advantageous means to reach and intervene among adolescents who use substances. Notably, social media advertising has been successfully used to recruit adolescent participants with substance use problems for trials not delivered by social media.[41] However, although some work suggests that Facebook may be an effective platform for substance use prevention,[42] and although 1 exploratory Tumblr-delivered intervention to young adults who smoke received encouraging qualitative feedback,[43] no studies to our knowledge have examined social media–delivered interventions designed to reduce substance use among adolescents. Thus, social media remains a largely understudied area that may be a potential platform from which to deliver interventions.

MULTISESSION INTERVENTIONS

Several controlled trials have evaluated multisession interventions for substance use among adolescents, all focused on universal samples regardless of risk level. Technology is seen as a scalable method for reducing risk among large samples of adolescents, most often in school or health care settings. This literature is reviewed here, breaking it into 2 unique subsections: multisession interventions in school settings, and multisession interventions using community samples.

Multisession Preventive Interventions in School Settings

Schools have long been the focus of universal programs designed to prevent risky substance use. As elsewhere, technology may facilitate the scalability and consistency of such efforts. Several trials in this area evaluate the Climate Schools program (**Fig. 2**), which consists of a series of in-school sessions in which adolescents in grades 8 through 10 first watch a 20-minute cartoon video, then engage in 20 minutes of classroom activities. Available modules, each consisting of 6 sessions, address alcohol, alcohol and cannabis together, or psychostimulants and cannabis.

Trials of the Climate Schools intervention show reliable increases in alcohol-related and/or cannabis-related knowledge. For example, Champion and colleagues[44] found that increases in knowledge at 6-month follow-up were strong (d = 0.67 for alcohol knowledge and 0.72 for cannabis knowledge). Controlled trials measuring alcohol use outcomes[44–48] all found reductions in alcohol use among students assigned to the intervention condition, although results for binge drinking outcomes were mixed. Of controlled trials measuring cannabis use outcomes, 2 found no advantage for the intervention condition,[44,49] and 1 found evidence of reduced use at the 6-month follow-up[50] but not at 12 months.[47]

Similar computer-delivered, school-based, multisession preventions tend to be shorter than the Climate Schools intervention. For example, the game-based, 3-session Alcohol Alert program[51] was tested in a cluster-randomized trial involving 34 classrooms including youth aged 15 to 19 years. At 4-month follow-up, binge drinking in the past 30 days was lower among youth assigned to the Alcohol Alert intervention. However, there were no between-group differences on secondary alcohol use outcomes, including number of drinks in the past week. Velicer and colleagues[52] found that a 5-session energy-balance intervention focused on physical activity, television watching, and diet had stronger effects on preventing alcohol use than a 5-session substance use prevention intervention. Similarly, the E-health4Uth prevention program, whether alone or in combination with a referral of at-risk youth to the school nurse, was not associated with lower rates of alcohol or drug use.[53] In a large cluster-randomized trial involving 23 schools and 3784 students, the Healthy School and Drugs prevention program[54] was not associated with any reductions in alcohol use, whether presented alone or in combination with school-based prevention activities (eg, a school-wide parent meeting, training for school staff). This trial also found no program-related effects on marijuana use.

Multisession Preventive Interventions with Community Samples

Schinke and colleagues[55] report that a program involving 9 Internet-based sessions of 45 minutes each, in a sample of 591 girls aged 11 to 13 years and their mothers, was associated with lower levels of alcohol and marijuana use at a 1-year follow-up. Schinke and colleagues[56] report similar results at a 2-year follow-up in a sample of 916 mother-daughter dyads. Also using a 9-session Internet-delivered intervention, Fang and colleagues [57] found positive results among a sample of 108 Asian-American girls aged 10 to 14 years. In addition, Schwinn and colleagues[41] report outcome results for RealTeen, a Web site with 9 separate online intervention sessions guided by an animated narrator. In a nationwide sample of 788 girls aged 13 to 14 years recruited via Facebook, the investigators report significant 1-year effects on binge drinking but not alcohol use frequency, marijuana use, or other drugs. In a subsequent article,[58] the investigators report significant effects on marijuana and

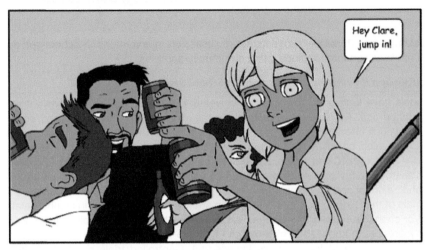

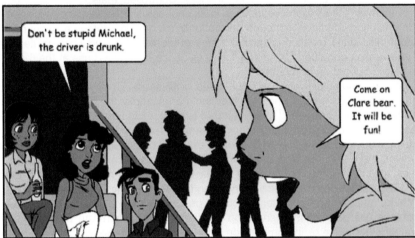

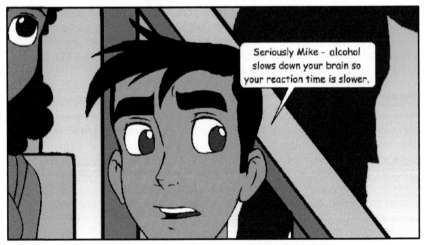

Fig. 2. Climate Schools program. (Images courtesy of the Climate Schools program, www. climateschools.com.au (Champion et al., 2016; Newton et al., 2009, 2010, 2014, 2018; Teeson et al., 2017).)

other drug use but not on alcohol use at 2 years, and no significant program effects on alcohol, marijuana, or other drugs at the 3-year follow-up.

SUMMARY

Technology-delivered interventions for adolescent substance use are becoming more widespread. These interventions have clear logistical advantages: they are inexpensive, easy to administer, and can be accessible at all times and from all locations. Technology-delivered interventions may be particularly well suited for adolescents, who are comfortable with technology and frequently use the Internet to obtain health information.[59]

Technology-delivered interventions come in several forms. Preventive interventions are the most prevalent form and aim to prevent the onset of substance use or reduce existing substance use. These interventions generally recruit participants from schools, primary care clinics, or the community. A second category of interventions focuses on reducing problem substance use in high-risk samples, such as in adolescents recruited from emergency departments who screen positive for risky substance use. In addition, a small group of studies has examined text-messaging interventions that target risky substance use and can be delivered either independently or in conjunction with Web-based or person-delivered interventions.

Evidence for the efficacy of technology-delivered interventions has been generally positive across a range of different substances (tobacco, alcohol, marijuana) and outcomes (eg, binge drinking, driving under the influence). Nonetheless, null findings are common, particularly from studies of multisession preventive interventions[53,54] and in studies focusing on drug rather than alcohol use. In addition, this literature faces important methodological challenges and limitations. For example, many studies in this area have high attrition rates, and few use advanced methods for handling missing data. Many studies fail to statistically correct for the use of multiple comparisons across multiple time points. In addition, studies in this area do not generally use biological methods (eg, urine drug screening) to confirm the presence/absence of substance use following interventions.

There are also several gaps/understudied areas in the literature on technology-delivered interventions among adolescents. In particular, no studies have examined social media–delivered interventions among adolescents, despite promising outcomes among college students. In addition, the literature on text-messaging interventions is small, despite the primacy of this communication method among adolescents. Future studies that focus on these areas, using large samples, appropriate statistical control, and biological verification of substance use, are needed. In sum, technology-delivered interventions show promise for reducing unhealthy substance use among adolescents. More research is needed to overcome methodological limitations and expand the literature to understudied areas.

REFERENCES

1. Johnston LD, Miech RA, O'Malley PM, et al. Monitoring the future national survey results on drug use, 1975-2017: overview, key findings on adolescent drug use. Available at: http://files.eric.ed.gov/fulltext/ED589762.pdf. Accessed August 28, 2019.
2. Vermeiren R, Schwab-Stone M, Deboutte D, et al. Violence exposure and substance use in adolescents: findings from three countries. Pediatrics 2003; 111(3):535–40.

3. Kelly AB, Evans-Whipp TJ, Smith R, et al. A longitudinal study of the association of adolescent polydrug use, alcohol use and high school non-completion. Addiction 2015;110(4):627–35.

4. Pardini D, White HR, Xiong SY, et al. Unfazed or dazed and confused: does early adolescent marijuana use cause sustained impairments in attention and academic functioning? J Abnorm Child Psychol 2015;43(7):1203–17.

5. Lynskey M, Hall W. The effects of adolescent cannabis use on educational attainment: a review. Addiction 2000;95(11):1621–30.

6. Guilamo-Ramos V, Litardo HA, Jaccard J. Prevention programs for reducing adolescent problem behaviors: Implications of the co-occurrence of problem behaviors in adolescence. J Adolesc Health 2005;36(1):82–6.

7. Miller PG, Butler E, Richardson B, et al. Relationships between problematic alcohol consumption and delinquent behaviour from adolescence to young adulthood. Drug Alcohol Rev 2016;35(3):317–25.

8. Bagge CL, Sher KJ. Adolescent alcohol involvement and suicide attempts: toward the development of a conceptual framework. Clin Psychol Rev 2008; 28(8):1283–96.

9. Schilling EA, Aseltine RH Jr, Glanovsky JL, et al. Adolescent alcohol use, suicidal ideation, and suicide attempts. J Adolesc Health 2009;44(4):335–41.

10. Sellers CM, Diaz-Valdes Iriarte A, Wyman Battalen A, et al. Alcohol and marijuana use as daily predictors of suicide ideation and attempts among adolescents prior to psychiatric hospitalization. Psychiatry Res 2019;273:672–7.

11. Hurd YL, Michaelides M, Miller ML, et al. Trajectory of adolescent cannabis use on addiction vulnerability. Neuropharmacology 2014;76 Pt B:416–24.

12. Silins E, Horwood LJ, Patton GC, et al. Young adult sequelae of adolescent cannabis use: an integrative analysis. Lancet Psychiatry 2014;1(4):286–93.

13. Lynskey MT, Heath AC, Bucholz KK, et al. Escalation of drug use in early-onset cannabis users vs co-twin controls. JAMA 2003;289(4):427–33.

14. Waldron HB, Turner CW. Evidence-based psychosocial treatments for adolescent substance abuse. J Clin Child Adolesc Psychol 2008;37(1):238–61.

15. Merikangas KR, He JP, Burstein M, et al. Service utilization for lifetime mental disorders in U.S. adolescents: results of the National Comorbidity Survey-Adolescent Supplement (NCS-A). J Am Acad Child Adolesc Psychiatry 2011; 50(1):32–45.

16. Miller WR, Sorensen JL, Selzer JA, et al. Disseminating evidence-based practices in substance abuse treatment: a review with suggestions. J Subst Abuse Treat 2006;31(1):25–39.

17. Resko SM, Walton MA, Chermack ST, et al. Therapist competence and treatment adherence for a brief intervention addressing alcohol and violence among adolescents. J Subst Abuse Treat 2012;42(4):429–37.

18. Toumbourou JW, Stockwell T, Neighbors C, et al. Interventions to reduce harm associated with adolescent substance use. Lancet 2007;369(9570):1391–401.

19. Delany PJ, Shields JJ, Willenbring ML, et al. Expanding the role of health services research as a tool to reduce the public health burden of alcohol use disorders. Subst Use Misuse 2008;43(12–13):1729–46.

20. Cole HA, Prassel HB, Carlson CR. A meta-analysis of computer-delivered drinking interventions for college students: a comprehensive review of studies from 2010 to 2016. J Stud Alcohol Drugs 2018;79(5):686–96.

21. Rooke S, Thorsteinsson E, Karpin A, et al. Computer-delivered interventions for alcohol and tobacco use: a meta-analysis. Addiction 2010;105(8):1381–90.

22. Cunningham RM, Chermack ST, Zimmerman MA, et al. Brief motivational interviewing intervention for peer violence and alcohol use in teens: one-year follow-up. Pediatrics 2012;129(6):1083–90.

23. Cunningham RM, Chermack ST, Ehrlich PF, et al. Alcohol interventions among underage drinkers in the ED: a randomized controlled trial. Pediatrics 2015;136(4): E783–93.

24. Walton MA, Chermack ST, Shope JT, et al. Effects of a brief intervention for reducing violence and alcohol misuse among adolescents a randomized controlled trial. JAMA 2010;304(5):527–35.

25. Walton MA, Bohnert K, Resko S, et al. Computer and therapist based brief interventions among cannabis-using adolescents presenting to primary care: one year outcomes. Drug Alcohol Depend 2013;132(3):646–53.

26. Arnaud N, Baldus C, Elgan TH, et al. Effectiveness of a web-based screening and fully automated brief motivational intervention for adolescent substance use: a randomized controlled trial. J Med Internet Res 2016;18(5):e103.

27. McCarty CA, Gersh E, Katzman K, et al. Screening and brief intervention with adolescents with risky alcohol use in school-based health centers: a randomized clinical trial of the Check Yourself tool. Subst Abus 2019. [Epub ahead of print].

28. Voogt CV, Kleinjan M, Poelen EA, et al. The effectiveness of a web-based brief alcohol intervention in reducing heavy drinking among adolescents aged 15-20 years with a low educational background: a two-arm parallel group cluster randomized controlled trial. BMC Public Health 2013;13:694.

29. Dawson DA, Grant BF, Stinson FS, et al. Effectiveness of the derived Alcohol Use Disorders Identification Test (AUDIT-C) in screening for alcohol use disorders and risk drinking in the US general population. Alcohol Clin Exp Res 2005;29(5): 844–54.

30. Knight JR, Sherritt L, Gibson EB, et al. Effect of computer-based substance use screening and brief behavioral counseling vs usual care for youths in pediatric primary care: a pilot randomized clinical trial. JAMA Netw Open 2019;2(6): e196258.

31. Doumas DM, Esp S, Turrisi R, et al. A test of the efficacy of a brief, web-based personalized feedback intervention to reduce drinking among 9th grade students. Addict Behav 2014;39(1):231–8.

32. Doumas DM, Esp S, Flay B, et al. A randomized controlled trial testing the efficacy of a brief online alcohol intervention for high school seniors. J Stud Alcohol Drugs 2017;78(5):706–15.

33. Doumas DM, Esp S. Reducing alcohol-related consequences among high school seniors: efficacy of a brief, web-based intervention. J Couns Dev 2019;97(1): 53–61.

34. Foundation SDSUR. Available at: http://www.echeckuptogo.com/usa/. Accessed August 21, 2019.

35. Knight JR, Kuzubova K, Csemy L, et al. Computer-facilitated screening and brief advice to reduce adolescents' heavy episodic drinking: a study in two countries. J Adolesc Health 2018;62(1):118–20.

36. Harris SK, Csemy L, Sherritt L, et al. Computer-facilitated substance use screening and brief advice for teens in primary care: an international trial. Pediatrics 2012;129(6):1072–82.

37. Teens, Social Media & Technology 2018 | Pew Research Center. Available at: https://www.pewinternet.org/2018/05/31/teens-social-media-technology-2018/. Accessed August 30, 2019.

38. How having smartphones (or not) shapes the way teens communicate | Pew Research Center. Available at: https://www.pewresearch.org/fact-tank/2015/08/20/how-having-smartphones-or-not-shapes-the-way-teens-communicate/. Accessed August 30, 2019.

39. Haug S, Paz Castro R, Kowatsch T, et al. Efficacy of a technology-based, integrated smoking cessation and alcohol intervention for smoking cessation in adolescents: results of a cluster-randomised controlled trial. J Subst Abuse Treat 2017;82:55–66.

40. Haug S, Paz Castro R, Kowatsch T, et al. Efficacy of a web- and text messaging-based intervention to reduce problem drinking in adolescents: results of a cluster-randomized controlled trial. J Consult Clin Psychol 2017;85(2):147–59.

41. Schwinn TM, Schinke SP, Hopkins J, et al. An online drug abuse prevention program for adolescent girls: posttest and 1-year outcomes. J Youth Adolesc 2018; 47(3):490–500.

42. Kousoulis AA, Kympouropoulos SP, Pouli DK, et al. From the classroom to facebook: a fresh approach for youth tobacco prevention. Am J Health Promot 2016; 30(5):390–3.

43. Jacobs MA, Cha S, Villanti AC, et al. Using tumblr to reach and engage young adult smokers: a proof of concept in context. Am J Health Behav 2016;40(1): 48–54.

44. Champion KE, Newton NC, Stapinski L, et al. A cross-validation trial of an Internet-based prevention program for alcohol and cannabis: preliminary results from a cluster randomised controlled trial. Aust N Z J Psychiatry 2016;50(1): 64–73.

45. Teesson M, Newton NC, Slade T, et al. Combined universal and selective prevention for adolescent alcohol use: a cluster randomized controlled trial. Psychol Med 2017;47(10):1761–70.

46. Newton NC, Conrod PJ, Rodriguez DM, et al. A pilot study of an online universal school-based intervention to prevent alcohol and cannabis use in the UK. BMJ open 2014;4(5):e004750.

47. Newton NC, Teesson M, Vogl LE, et al. Internet-based prevention for alcohol and cannabis use: final results of the Climate Schools course. Addiction 2010;105(4): 749–59.

48. Newton NC, Vogl LE, Teesson M, et al. CLIMATE schools: alcohol module: cross-validation of a school-based prevention programme for alcohol misuse. Aust N Z J Psychiatry 2009;43(3):201–7.

49. Newton NC, Teesson M, Mather M, et al. Universal cannabis outcomes from the Climate and Preventure (CAP) study: a cluster randomised controlled trial. Subst Abuse Treat Prev Policy 2018;13(1):34.

50. Newton NC, Andrews G, Teesson M, et al. Delivering prevention for alcohol and cannabis using the Internet: a cluster randomised controlled trial. Prev Med 2009; 48(6):579–84.

51. Jander A, Crutzen R, Mercken L, et al. Effects of a web-based computer-tailored game to reduce binge drinking among dutch adolescents: a cluster randomized controlled trial. J Med Internet Res 2016;18(2):e29.

52. Velicer WF, Redding CA, Paiva AL, et al. Multiple behavior interventions to prevent substance abuse and increase energy balance behaviors in middle school students. Transl Behav Med 2013;3(1):82–93.

53. Bannink R, Broeren S, Joosten-van Zwanenburg E, et al. Effectiveness of a Web-based tailored intervention (E-health4Uth) and consultation to promote adolescents' health: randomized controlled trial. J Med Internet Res 2014;16(5):e143.

54. Malmberg M, Kleinjan M, Overbeek G, et al. Effectiveness of the 'Healthy School and Drugs' prevention programme on adolescents' substance use: a randomized clustered trial. Addiction 2014;109(6):1031–40.

55. Schinke SP, Fang L, Cole KC. Preventing substance use among adolescent girls: 1-year outcomes of a computerized, mother-daughter program. Addict Behav 2009;34(12):1060–4.

56. Schinke SP, Fang L, Cole KC. Computer-delivered, parent-involvement intervention to prevent substance use among adolescent girls. Prev Med 2009;49(5): 429–35.

57. Fang L, Schinke SP, Cole KC. Preventing substance use among early Asian-American adolescent girls: initial evaluation of a web-based, mother-daughter program. J Adolesc Health 2010;47(5):529–32.

58. Schwinn TM, Schinke SP, Keller B, et al. Two- and three-year follow-up from a gender-specific, web-based drug abuse prevention program for adolescent girls. Addict Behav 2019;93:86–92.

59. Gray NJ, Klein JD, Noyce PR, et al. The Internet: a window on adolescent health literacy. J Adolesc Health 2005;37(3):243.

Moving?

Make sure your subscription moves with you!

To notify us of your new address, find your **Clinics Account Number** (located on your mailing label above your name), and contact customer service at:

Email: journalscustomerservice-usa@elsevier.com

800-654-2452 (subscribers in the U.S. & Canada)
314-447-8871 (subscribers outside of the U.S. & Canada)

Fax number: 314-447-8029

Elsevier Health Sciences Division
Subscription Customer Service
3251 Riverport Lane
Maryland Heights, MO 63043

*To ensure uninterrupted delivery of your subscription, please notify us at least 4 weeks in advance of move.

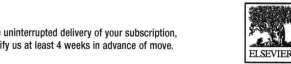

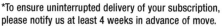